Performance and Dementia

"This is a vibrant and important book that weaves together themes of performance, creativity and care with an instinctive eye for ethnographic detail. Hatton's writing is alert and precise, capturing the tensions in negotiating theatre practice in care environments. The book provokes new thinking on established concepts in the arts, dementia and well-being discourse, and argues for a new approach governed by a situational understanding of relationality between people living with dementia and the spaces they occupy. The writing is accessible, complex and beautifully evocative."

—Professor Michael Balfour, *University of New South Wales, Sydney*

Nicky Hatton

Performance and Dementia

A Cultural Response to Care

palgrave
macmillan

Nicky Hatton
York, UK

ISBN 978-3-030-51076-3 ISBN 978-3-030-51077-0 (eBook)
https://doi.org/10.1007/978-3-030-51077-0

Cover image by Jules Dorey Richmond, inspired by The Storybox Project. Storybox Project photography by Roshana Rubin-Mayhew.

This Palgrave Macmillan imprint is published by the registered company Springer Nature Switzerland AG.
The registered company address is: Gewerbestrasse 11, 6330 Cham, Switzerland

To Laurie and Nina, with love

Preface

1994, Headingley, Leeds

I am eight years old and attending primary school in Leeds. It is December and Year 4 class have been rehearsing Christmas carols all week. This morning we are due to perform to residents at a care home down the road. It is a care home that I walk past every morning on my way to school but have never really noticed before. We are nervous and excited as we trundle down the street, bundled up in our winter hats and coats. We have been practising all week and are hyped up at the prospect of an audience. When we arrive at the care home we are shown into a lounge which feels stuffy and airless. The residents are sitting in rows of high-backed armchairs which have deep red upholstery and white antimacassars. I don't remember much about the concert itself apart from the fact that I feel itchy and uncomfortable in my woolly hat. One moment stands out though. About halfway through the concert, a male resident beckons over a member of care staff and requests *Hark the Herald Angels Sing*. There is a slightly awkward moment. We haven't rehearsed that one so we plough on with *Good King Wenceslas* instead. About a verse in the man stands and proceeds, with some effort, to pick up his chair from underneath him. Slowly and deliberately, he turns it around 180 degrees so that he has his back to us. I'm shocked and leave with the impression that old people in care homes are quite frightening. The moment stays with me over the next few days as I walk past the care home on my way to school and peer solemnly up at the net-curtained windows.

2011, Swiss Cottage, London

It is 17 years before I have my next experience of a care home. I am working as the Creative Learning Practitioner for Hampstead Theatre, running scriptwriting projects in local schools. We have just been told that the local authority are pulling their financial support for our programme and we are working flat out to secure emergency funding. It is around this time that I receive a phone call from a care home on the same street as the theatre. The man on the other end of the phone is the activity coordinator and wants to know if there is 'anything we can do for the residents', most of whom are living with late stage dementia. Again, I realise that I have walked past this care home several times a week on my way to workshops but never noticed it before. It also occurs to me that I have had no experience of dementia, in a personal or a professional capacity. We agree to go along one morning to meet the residents.

The care home is a large converted Victorian house which on first glance looks like the rest of the houses on the street. As we approach the front door though I see that it is has a number of locks and keypads and a buzzer entry system. After a few minutes of buzzing and waiting we are shown in by the activity coordinator. Brightly coloured murals adorn the corridor and there is large red post box painted at one end with a tray for residents to put letters in. We are shown into a lounge where the residents are sat in armchairs facing the television. The activity coordinator turns the TV down a fraction and addresses them loudly: 'There's two ladies come from the theatre who want to talk to you'. A couple of the residents look at us, others continue to watch television. We introduce ourselves but it is difficult to be heard over the noise of the television and we are conscious that we are interrupting. We decide to talk to some of the residents individually and I crouch down awkwardly next to two women who are sat together. I'm not sure what to say so I attempt polite conversation, telling them about Hampstead Theatre and asking them about themselves. I ask 'did you grow up in Camden?' One of the women smiles at me and nods. The other looks at me with a slightly anxious expression. I realise that I have made a mistake and that by asking her questions about the past, I may be putting pressure on her to recall things that she doesn't remember. Feeling foolish, I change tact, and compliment her on her skirt, which has a dark print of flowers and birds. She looks at her skirt and smiles at me. We sit in silence for a while. I'm not sure where to go next. We leave a bit deflated and unsure of how to proceed.

A few days later my manager tells me that she called the care home and told them that we couldn't work with them this time. She doesn't think that our scriptwriting model can be adapted to fit the needs of the residents and in our current financial circumstances, we don't have the capacity to develop new work. I understand the reasons behind her decision, but I can't help feeling we have let them down. I am left with lots of questions. Are there any theatre practitioners working in care homes? What sort of work is taking place? Is it possible to make theatre with people who are experiencing late stage dementia? How might I go about adapting my own practice? Over the next few weeks I start to do some digging.

2013, Dalston, London

Two years later I'm standing in the dining room of 20–26 Mildmay Park, a care home in North-East London, with a camera, a notepad and a measuring tape. Accompanying me is activity coordinator Marian, whom I have been shadowing for the past few weeks and a resident called Lottie. At the other end of the room care staff crowd around a large TV watching coverage of Nelson Mandela's funeral. I have started a PhD about theatre in care homes. We are discussing the possibility of a site-specific project that will take place in the dining room and I'm excited. I want to explore how we can use theatre to make it into a more homely space. However, volunteering at the care home has thrown up a lot of practical questions and I'm finding it difficult to visualise what the project will look like. How will I run workshops with the residents when the space is constantly in use for mealtimes and other activities? How will I minimise the disruption that these workshops create in the dining room? How will we address the aesthetic challenges of the space; the noise from the adjoining kitchen, the heavy tables and chairs that can't be moved easily, the health and safety regulations which restricts the use of electrical equipment, the flimsy curtains that won't allow the space to go dark?

Over the next few weeks I visit Mildmay on a number of occasions to try and get a sense of how it will work. I have lunch with the residents, join the weekly quiz team and attend a concert of Christmas carols. I serve drinks at a cocktail party and help the activity coordinator to move residents to and from different sites. After a while I become familiar with the daily schedule for mealtimes, activities and trips to and from day centres. I learn a little about the relationships that residents have with each other and with the different spaces in the home. I find out for example, that

Amir likes to watch *Columbo* at 4 pm every day in the lounge as this is a time when he is unlikely to be disturbed. I become familiar with the care home's sensory properties: the buzz of the door entry system, the smell of the dining room and the dim lighting in the corridors. The more time I spend there, the more intrigued I am by the care home as a community which has its own particular routines and customs. I realise that my interest has shifted from the impact of theatre on the care home to a creative interest in Mildmay itself. Rather than trying to work around the routines of the home, I am curious about finding an approach which acknowledges them, or in some way incorporates them into the creative process. This relationship between creative practice and the care environment is at the heart of this book.

York, UK Nicky Hatton

Acknowledgements

I would like to thank the residents and staff of 20–26 Mildmay Park in London who inspired this book and made it possible. Thank you for welcoming me so warmly into your home and for encouraging me to think about creativity in new ways. Particular thanks is due to Marian Howell, Mildmay's Activities' Officer, for her support and insights. I am grateful to Notting Hill Genesis for enabling me to work with Mildmay, and to all the participants who took part in workshops and conversations. Thank you to former MA students Sara Athens, Stella Nouli and Jessie Sherman from the Royal Central School of Speech and Drama, and to Jamie Flockton who collaborated with me on much of the practice.

I am extremely thankful to Helen Nicholson for her guidance and ongoing support as my PhD supervisor and beyond. I am also very grateful to my second supervisor Tony Evans, and to the following practitioners and scholars who generously shared their ideas and practice: Nicky Taylor, Jayne Lloyd, David Grindley, Ben Owen, James Thompson, Liz Postlethwaite, Lowri Evans and Sara Cocker.

Thank you to the Taking Part team at the Young Vic Theatre for helping me to access their production of *Turning a Little Further*: particularly Imogen Brodie, Laura Keefe and Lily Einhorn. I am extremely grateful to performers Boma Braide, Hilary Friend and Jill Reyes who kindly took part in interviews and shared their time very generously, offering a great deal of insight into the lives of unpaid carers.

I am grateful to the Faculty of Arts at the University of Winchester who granted me research leave to write this book, and to my former colleagues—Marilena Zaroulia, Marianne Sharp, and Helen Grime, who offered support along the way. I would also like to thank my new colleagues at York St John University, particularly Matthew Reason, for supporting me during the final stages of publication. I am grateful to the Arts and Humanities Research Council for funding my PhD studentship so that I could conduct this research.

Thank you to the following people for granting permission for me to use photos of their work: Melanie Wilson, Monika Chimerlz, Imogen Brodie, Liz Postlethwaite, Nicky Taylor and Pete Grogan.

Finally, thanks to my family and friends for their support: in particular, to my husband Alex for his gentle encouragement, to my sister Rebecca, and to my mum Kate for looking after Laurie so that I could finish the book.

A shorter version of Chap. 7 has been previously published and appears in a themed edition of Research in Drama Education on *Theatre, Dementia and Relationality*. I would like to thank Taylor and Francis for their permission to re-use this work here.

Residents' names have been anonymised in this book to protect their identities. This is with the exception of one resident, Lydia, who chose to appear in a photograph alongside the work she had made. In this instance, consent was kindly granted by Lydia's family on her behalf, for her name and photo to be used in Chap. 6. I am grateful to Lydia and her family for allowing me to do this.

Contents

List of Figures

CHAPTER 1

Introduction: Performance, Creativity and Care

Working with the System

> Systems have their own dramaturgy, and you can think about intervening, or you can think about embedding or blending around, or working within. All too often we think about whatever system we're landing in as the thing you have to negotiate in order to do the thing we really want to do … but you have to find a way to work with the system, dramaturgically. (Rohd in Basting et al. 2016, p. 39)

In 2009, the American theatre director Michael Rohd began a new project with Sojourn Theatre, the Portland-based ensemble that he had founded a decade earlier. The Homeric-inspired *Finding Penelope* took place in a large retirement community and engaged care staff, theatre practitioners, dancers and residents from different parts of the care home. The project took place over two years across different sites, rehearsing in dining rooms, lounge spaces and residents' bedrooms, before leading the audience in a promenade performance around the care home. It is significant, not least because it was the first professional theatre production to be made in a care setting, but because of its aim to work collaboratively with staff and residents. Sojourn have a history of making site-specific performances and work on what they describe as a continuum of 'social/civic practice' (Ibid., p. 17). The social, in their terms, refers to work that is initiated by an artistic desire to 'explore/create a conceptual event or series of moments' (Ibid.), whereas the civic aspect of their practice is

N. Hatton, *Performance and Dementia*,
https://doi.org/10.1007/978-3-030-51077-0_1

concerned with making work 'in response to the goals of non-arts partners' (Ibid., p. 18). Working with a care community blurred the distinctions between these two types of practice. Reflecting on some of the challenges of getting started, Rohd describes how their intentions shifted as a result of rehearsing in communal spaces. Initially, the routine of the care home was perceived as a system to be negotiated and overcome in order to get down to the 'real work' of making the play. However, Rohd and his colleagues soon realised that any meaningful collaboration would involve working with this system 'dramaturgically'.

Rohd's observations resonate with my own experiences of making performance in care homes in the UK. I often find myself working with residents in communal spaces where there are other activities taking place. These have included structured activities such as mealtimes and activity programmes, and unstructured events such as napping and watching television. Bringing arts projects into care settings inevitably disrupts these activities and running creative sessions alongside them can be challenging. Introducing new activities while respecting residents' privacy and the routines of the care home requires sensitivity and flexibility. While it can be difficult to work within the institutional structures of a care home, there is an opportunity to pay attention to its routines and rhythms, and to develop modes of practice which are collaborative and responsive.

This is a book about how participatory arts, and performance in particular, can change the way we think about dementia care and some of the environments in which it takes place. Drawing on my own practice, and performance projects that are taking place in care homes in the UK, it explores some of the challenges and opportunities associated with making performance in care settings. Rather than focusing on the transformative potential of the arts in dementia care, it asks how artists can engage with the different types of relationships that exist in a care community. These include the relationships that residents and staff have with each other as well as relationships they have with the home itself. Exploring the intersection between participatory arts and the everyday creativity of a care home, my aim is to generate insights into the cultural importance of the arts in care homes, and to promote dementia care as a relational practice. I also hope to shed light on the intrinsic creativity of caregiving and how principles and practices of care can inform theatre and performance in diverse ways. The book is intended as a resource for the growing number of artists who are developing work in, with, and in response to care homes, as well as care professionals who are interested in bringing creativity into their working lives.

When I started working in care homes in 2012, 'arts in dementia care' was emerging as a field of participatory arts practice in the UK. Since then, the scale and variety of practices that take place has increased significantly and there are now more artists working in care homes than ever before. The 'Arts and Older People in Care' grant, launched by Arts Council England and the Baring Foundation in 2012 was 'the largest level of creative investment in care homes ever seen in the UK' (Baring Foundation 2018, p. 21), and indicative of a shift away from the arts as a health intervention towards creative practice which demonstrated artistic quality and innovation. The criteria that was stipulated for this grant included 'providing access to high quality arts experiences', 'establish[ing] a series of sustainable, exemplar programmes of arts and engagement activity', stretch[ing] aspiration, and 'showcas[ing] artistic excellence in residential care settings (Arts Council 2013, p. 4). This commitment to artistic excellence points to the shifting priorities of arts funders in supporting high quality arts practices in care settings—a priority which is shared by many performance practitioners. Between 2015 and 2017, the intergenerational charity Magic Me organised a series of residencies for performance artists in collaboration with the care home provider Anchor. The aim was to 'open the doors on new possibilities for care homes as places where inspiring and important art is created' (Begault et al. 2017, p. 4). The artists involved; Punchdrunk Enrichment, Upswing, Lois Weaver and Duckie—are all practitioners with an international artistic profile as well as a commitment to socially engaged practice. The contemporary focus of these residencies, which included immersive installations, circus and cabaret are indicative of this shift towards experimentation and artistic quality. Performance practitioners are increasingly exploring the aesthetic possibilities of collaboration and raising the bar on the artistic experiences available to residents.

The performances explored in this book operate within a wider context of participatory arts and dementia, in the UK and internationally. In the United States, for example, the development of participatory performance for people with dementia has been pioneered by the playwright Anne Basting, whose improvisational *Timeslips* approach has supported the participation of people at the later stages of dementia.[1] In the UK, Age Exchange Theatre Trust, a company with a long-term history of working with older people, have expanded and adapted their reminiscence theatre work so that it can be accessed more easily by those living with dementia.[2] Rather than offering an overview of this expanding field, the book poses critical questions about theatre and performance's role in care environments. It does not attempt to capture the spectrum of performance work that is taking place. Rather, it makes a case for performative approaches that are sensory and experiential. By focusing on specific projects in care homes in the UK, my aim is to examine closely the creative potential of these institutional spaces and to understand how performance practitioners respond to the particular challenges and opportunities of working with an eldercare community.

A common difficulty of collaborating with care homes is that care staff rarely have the opportunity to take part. This is due to the volume of their workloads and the demands of a task-oriented care system which allows little time for activities that fall outside the boundaries of primary care. Rota systems often mean different working patterns each week, making it difficult for carers to commit to a regular timeslot. While every partnership is different, this was an issue in many of the projects discussed here which, despite efforts to include them, featured little regular participation from care staff. This absence of carers poses a particular challenge to a book about performance and care. It is difficult to see how creative approaches might be embedded within caring relationships after an arts project has finished if carers have not been involved. However, it is also an invitation for artists to think about other ways of working with carers so that they can access arts activities, and for their knowledge and experiences to be built into a creative project at different stages. The final chapter of this book is a response to this challenge and explores some of the imaginative ways that performance practitioners are trying to work with carers in light of these restrictions.

Beyond a contextual consideration, the book does not address the creative and relational acts of care that take place between people with dementia and their carers outside of formal care settings. This is beyond its scope. However, it acknowledges this richer context and the fact that the majority of people with dementia are still cared for by friends and family members at home. While the focus of the book is the creative potential of formal care spaces, I hope that the connections it promotes between creativity and care will be of relevance to those engaged in caring roles at home, which are unpaid and often go unnoticed. In particular, I hope that the focus on performances made by unpaid carers in the final chapter will offer some insight into how theatre can raise the status and visibility of carers—both inside and outside of formal care settings.

Defining Performance

I am writing at a time when participatory theatre and performance are being reconceptualised as ecologies of practice which continually shift and develop, rather than as a static discipline of participatory work. In their book *Critical Perspectives on Applied Theatre,* Jenny Hughes and Helen Nicholson outline some of the priorities and themes that are emerging as practitioners and researchers negotiate, among other things, environmental concerns. These include 'theatre's relationship to temporality and cultural memory, the politics of place, environment and attachment, and the material and relational dimensions of human and non-human agency' (Hughes and Nicholson 2016, p. 2). Their attention to human and non-human agency echo the concerns of this book, which calls for a relational approach, both in the way that we care for people with dementia and how we approach performance practice in care homes. In Chap. 3, I propose a new approach to dementia care which is inspired by posthumanism and the relational exchanges that take place between people and care spaces. My approach is informed by this shift in attention in applied theatre research towards ecology: what Hughes and Nicholson describe as a 'productive relationship ... between human agency and the agentic capacities of the material world' (Ibid., p. 9). The principles of posthumanism are used throughout the book to illuminate the potential of performance practices that are inspired by the wider material environment.

Alongside this shift in applied theatre research is a move towards care as an artistic and participatory concern. In his article *Towards an aesthetics of care*, James Thompson considers the 'radical potential' of placing community-engaged arts work 'within the framework of care' (Thompson 2015, p. 432). He recalls a personal experience of looking after a Congolese colleague who had been injured during a massacre in the DR Congo. After the attack, the colleague travelled to Manchester to receive medical treatment and lived for a while with Thompson and his family. Reflecting on his friend's recovery, Thompson draws a connection between the intimacy and beauty that was involved in one-to-one encounters with his physiotherapist and the qualities of inter-human relationships that can emerge through community-based performance. Though he is writing about a different caring context, his call for an 'aesthetic turn in care studies' (Ibid.) resonates within this book. Thompson's emphasis on the relational process of artistic creation raises questions about how arts practitioners working in care settings might support caregiving as a creative endeavour in the context of a task-oriented care sector. The term 'aesthetics of care' is an invitation to consider what is radical about theatre and performance in helping us think about care as a creative and reciprocal process. However, it also asks what performance makers can learn from care homes and how these experiences translate to performance elsewhere.

This book discusses examples of theatre and performance practice. Though it is at times concerned with theatrical experiences, I have chosen to use the word 'performance' in its title, firstly because it encompasses the cross-disciplinary nature of the practice, which includes theatre, storytelling, visual arts, sound, film, music and installation work. The hybrid nature of the work can also be understood in terms of Shannon Jackson's 'widened discourse of performance' (Jackson 2011, p. 2), which she outlines in her book *Social Works*. This is partly because of its interdisciplinarity but also because the creative work discussed is concerned with her concept of interdependence. Questions of the aesthetic and the social wrestle in care homes as they do in *Social Works*, because a care home is, quite literally, a site where 'aesthetic and social provocations coincide' (Ibid., p. 5). Arts projects usually take place in communal spaces, which are used for a range of social purposes. An artist is an outsider, an intruder to the social life of a care home which has its own routines and customs. As I explore in Chap. 6, participation in a performance project can reveal things about the social dynamics of a care home and the position of residents within its community. It creates opportunities for 'inter-dependent social imagining(s)' (Ibid., p. 14), by putting residents and artists in situations where they are working collaboratively together. Jackson's definition of performance as a 'series of supporting relations' (Ibid., p. 42) is integral to my framing of creativity in an institutional care context, and to understanding the particular contribution of people with dementia to a performance-making process.

Furthermore, the term 'performance' is applicable to the myriad creative ways in which people with dementia negotiate social situations in care homes, an idea that is explored in detail in Chap. 6 through an exploration of social networks, and in Chap. 7 through Tim Ingold and Elizabeth Hallam's (Hallam and Ingold 2008) concept of 'cultural improvisation'. The notion of performance in everyday life, as advanced by Erving Goffman (1990) and Richard Schechner (2003) takes on an interesting dimension in a dementia care setting where residents are often required to improvise their way through social encounters. Schechner interprets Goffman's theory of performance as a 'mode of behaviour' and a 'quality that can occur in any situation rather than a fenced off genre' (Schechner 2003, p. 22). His interpretation is instructive in understanding the type of creativity that occurs as part of daily life in a care home as residents attune to new social situations. In Chap. 7, I argue that the repetition of personal routines by people with dementia is a type of creative performance which can enable them to re-create a sense of home. Utilising performance as an 'inclusive term' (ibid., p. xvii) enables me to distinguish between the creative practice of artists and people living with dementia, and crucially, where these two types of performance meet in the middle.

Finally, my preference for the term 'performance' over 'theatre' is because the creative works explored in this book tend to prioritise the performance event and its aesthetic effects over theatrical narratives. In this sense, they are largely experiential rather than representational. The purpose here is not to avoid theatrical discourse but to emphasise a connection between experiential performance and the creative affordances of a care environment. Furthermore, text-based theatre which uses dialogue, action and plot is not always appropriate for people living with dementia, who can struggle to make sense of a linear narrative. At times this book borrows from the vocabulary of postdramatic theatre to articulate scenarios where performances might be 'helpfully defamiliarising' (Jackson 2011, p. 3). In Chap. 3, for example, I explore how dramaturgical approaches such as episodic structures, fragmented narratives and absurdist repetitions can offer a more authentic means of representing the lived experience of dementia, as well as making theatre-going a more accessible experience. Concepts of experiential performance, therefore, are central to the idea of 'dementia-friendly theatre' and in understanding how performance practitioners can engage creatively with a care environment.

Interdisciplinary Connections

Exploring the intersection between performance, creativity and care is an interdisciplinary endeavour that sits, sometimes awkwardly, between the fields of theatre, performance, health, disability, ageing and dementia studies. The terms 'arts and older people', and 'arts and dementia' are increasingly being applied in the Global North to describe research that enhances our understanding of the connections between ageing and creativity. Arts and Dementia has become established as a field of research in its own right. It incorporates diverse methodological approaches, often bringing research teams together across disciplines. Research that comes under this banner ranges from quantitative studies that aim to understand the health benefits of the arts in dementia care (Keating et al. 2018), to Social Return on Investment analyses of arts groups (Jones et al. 2014), and arts-led studies which examine creative approaches and aesthetic outcomes (Nicholson et al. 2014; Harris 2013). These studies pose different questions about the value of the work. In a publication about the 'challenge of cultural gerontology', Julia Twigg and Wendy Martin remark that 'arts and humanities scholars have brought not just new subject areas [to ageing studies] but also new epistemologies and methodologies' (Twigg and Martin 2015, p. 354). Their observation suggests that there is more to be understood about the specific contribution of arts-based research methods to gerontological research, especially when the research is about older people's engagement with the arts. As discussed in the next chapter, there is a burgeoning understanding that arts-based research methods can capture something that other research methods cannot, particularly when the participants may not be able to participate in formal research processes.

My understanding of a cultural response has been shaped by evolving theories of caregiving, offered through social work, dementia studies and cultural gerontology. Cultural gerontologists who examine the social and cultural dimensions of ageing raise important questions for performance scholars and practitioners as to how factors such as age, gender, race, disability and class are played out across the social space of a care home. A cultural or creative response to care must acknowledge that a care home community is made up of a broad demographic of older people who are ageing differently. There is also much that can be gained from using a performative lens to examine care spaces. While cultural gerontologists have pointed to the potential of arts-based methodologies in attending to the 'complex interplay between the body and its social and cultural constitution of age' (Ibid., p. 355), this is not something which has been explored in the context of arts in care homes. This book attends to this gap, opening a new critical space in which the social and cultural dynamics of dementia care are explored through the lens of performance.

Overview of This Book

This book is structured in two parts. Part I, *A Cultural Response*, considers the creative value of performance in care settings and how it can change the way we think about dementia care. It explores how non-naturalistic, experiential approaches to performance-making can support dementia care as a relational practice, attending to the wider care giving environment, as well as relationships between people with dementia and their carers.

Chapter 2 contextualises the book within the expanding field of arts and dementia care. It traces how the field developed in the UK in response to government policies such as the National Dementia Strategy (Department of Health 2009) and The Prime Minister's Challenge on Dementia (Department of Health 2012), which sought to improve quality of life. It argues that our understanding about the role of the arts in dementia care has been shaped by a 'wellbeing agenda', in which the value of an arts project is measured chiefly against its potential to improve the wellbeing of participants. It suggests that the concept of wellbeing is inappropriate for people with dementia, because of its associations with idealised forms of citizenship, which people with dementia do not conform to.

The remainder of the chapter sets out the need for a cultural response. It considers the crisis-status of dementia in the West, how connections between memory and selfhood are culturally ingrained, and how dementia is in part socially constructed by our fears about ageing and memory loss. It considers how participatory arts have the capacity to respond to these fears on a cultural level by supporting concepts of memory and selfhood which are based on interdependence and relationality, rather than independence and autonomy.

Chapter 3 looks at how theatre and performance makers are responding to dementia and the emergence of a dementia-friendly theatre movement. It explores how representations of dementia on stage are beginning to shift from the experience of carers, to that of those living with dementia, and how people with dementia are being involved in theatre-making processes. Analysing key examples of collaborative performance work, it looks at some of the productive ways that people with dementia are challenging processes of creative production. Foregrounding the relationship between access and aesthetics, it explores the specific contribution of dementia-friendly theatre to the growing neurodiversity and performance sector by re-framing theatre-going as an interdependent and vulnerable experience.

Building on these creative approaches, Chap. 4 explores the possibilities of a relational approach to dementia care which is inspired by posthumanism. It argues that dementia care needs to be thought of within a broader relational context in which caregiving relationships and the physical and atmospheric properties of a care environment are interrelated. Inspired by examples of ecological performance, it imagines an approach to participatory performance in care homes which supports this type of dementia care in practice. Namely, an approach which attends to the environmental elements of a care home and the way they are encountered through the body.

Part II, *Performance and the Care Environment*, offers a practice-based discussion on performance-making in care homes. It is illustrated with examples from my own work at a care home called 20–26 Mildmay Park in London, as well as the work of Manchester-based community arts company Small Things. Each chapter relates to performance-making and a specific aspect of the care environment.

Chapter 5 considers how performance practitioners can be inspired by a care home's aural properties, and how the sounds of a care home may be 're-imagined' or perceived differently through creative practice. It offers an analysis of a sound installation that I created with residents over a six-week period, which was inspired by the aural properties of the dining room. Drawing on the philosopher Gaston Bachelard's work on the re-imagining of everyday spaces, it argues that sound can establish a sense of place in a care home, as well as connecting residents to other significant times and places from their pasts.

Chapter 6 looks at the social environment of the care home, exploring the relationship between community, taste and participation. It explores how residents express their personal tastes through participatory arts projects, and how these tastes are negotiated in relation to each other. The first part of the chapter looks at taste and material culture. It reflects on an interior design workshop that I ran with care home residents, in order to consult them about the redecoration of the care home. Revisiting sociologist Dick Hebdige's (1979) work on style and subculture, and Grayson Perry's work on domestic taste, it considers the significance of taste in a care home, where opportunities to display decorative and homely objects are restricted.

The second part of this chapter explores cultural taste in the context of a popular music project. It explores what the expression of taste in a creative context reveals about the social environment of a care community. Participation in an arts project can increase opportunities for residents to express their tastes, but it can also highlight differences, particularly in relation to age, class, education and cultural background. Reflecting on the project, it considers how the cultural tastes of care home residents are evolving with the ageing population, and the aesthetic implications this has for arts practices in care homes.

Chapter 7 is about collaboration. It explores the relationship between creativity and care in STORYBOX, an improvisational storytelling programme for people with dementia. Using concepts of domestic creativity and cultural improvisation, it explores some of the ways in which creativity occurs as residents negotiate everyday life in a care home, and how artists might find ways of engaging with it. Rather than thinking of performance practices in care homes in terms of their transformative potential, it rethinks collaboration between artists and people with dementia as two sets of creative practice meeting in the middle.

Chapter 8, *A Caring Effect*, considers the wider implications of this book. Firstly, it considers the legacy of performance projects for care homes in the context of the Arts Council's *Arts in Care Homes* programme, which 'sought to develop a more embedded, cross-sector approach' (Baring Foundation 2018, p. 5) to collaboration between care homes and arts organisations. Reflecting on the practice discussed in the book, it explores some of the problems of capturing the 'impact' of an arts project when residents may not remember it and care staff may not have taken part. It argues that concepts of ephemerality and affect might offer a more appropriate means of interpreting the changes that can occur through performance practice than frameworks that try to measure change in quantifiable ways. Addressing the challenge of working with carers, it goes on to suggest some ways that artists might incorporate the specialist knowledge of carers into creative practice and draw on their expertise when planning a project. It identifies some opportunities for introducing creative activities within the daily practices of caregiving and explore how online and virtual learning programmes might also enable carers to deliver arts activities themselves.

The book concludes by considering the contribution of carers to contemporary performance practice more broadly. Focusing on *Turning a Little Further*, a Young Vic Theatre production which featured carers as performers, it explores how caring attributes can be embedded into a performance process and generate new ways of working. It considers the wider significance of care as a way of working within the theatre industry and how different manifestations of 'performing care' might counter a more damaging culture of #selfcare within a younger generation of performance makers.

Much of the practice explored in the book has emerged from my own performance work in care settings. As a practitioner-researcher, I had the opportunity to work with one care home over an 18-month period. This enabled me to explore, test and develop many of the theoretical and creative approaches discussed in the book. It also means that this project has been a rather personal journey, which has challenged my own attitudes towards ageing, capacity and creativity. I began this work with some trepidation in my late 20s with no personal or professional experience of dementia. This trepidation was shaped, to some extent, by a fear of care homes that began in young childhood. However, I was plagued by a much more immediate fear, described in the prologue, that I would arrive and not know what to *do*. I realised fairly quickly that the work I was about to embark on required a very different approach from the participatory work that I had done in schools, or indeed other institutional settings. Learning how to *be* in this environment with residents, and identity opportunities for creativity and participation, required a particular type of attention to small, everyday types of artistry. This tension between doing and being is an important part of the attunement that is discussed in Chap. 6 when I write about slowing down and reconfiguring our sense of pace. It is also something I am learning about in another area of my life. Since I started writing, I have embarked on a new caring role as a parent. This experience is teaching me something about everyday acts of care and the creativity required in balancing caring responsibilities with those of an early career researcher. Over the last three years, the 'thinking work' that previously characterised my day-to-day working life has competed with a more embodied, intuitive type of role. Furthermore, my connection to care homes has taken on a more personal association since my grandma moved into one. It is now that of a visitor/family member rather than an arts practitioner. To my grandma, the idea of taking part in an arts project, or indeed any form of 'organised fun', is a cringeworthy prospect, and she is a reminder that care home residents may have little choice in whether an arts project takes place at their home. My experiences support Thompson's claim that the 'professional' cannot be sustained ethically without a commitment to the potential for it to blur dynamically with the personal' (Thompson 2015, p. 432). I am reminded that the intimate dimensions of caring relationships that exist outside of theatre practice and academic research inevitably shapes the way in which we move towards an 'aesthetics of care' in our 'professional' lives.

The question of choice also highlights the ethical complexities of conducting participatory research with older people in care homes. The community at Mildmay Park is made up of residents with cognitive differences and a spectrum of communication needs. Some of these residents were able to give informed consent to participate and others were not. In instances where a resident was not able to give consent, advice was sought from family members or care staff who knew them well and were able to advise on the appropriateness of their participation. However, the capacity of certain residents to give consent would sometimes fluctuate, depending on the day.

In her article about the politics of trust in Drama Education, Helen Nicholson argues that trust is dependent on context and must be 'continually negotiated and re-negotiated in action' (Nicholson 2002, p. 81). Her argument is pertinent to conducting research with people who are living with dementia, and specifically, the way in consent needed to be treated as an ongoing process in this research. Some residents would choose to participate in a workshop session one week but opt out during other times. In these instances, their decision was always respected, along with the assurance that they were welcome to re-join the group at any point if they wanted to. For the residents who had dementia, preferences to opt out were sometimes harder to identify and required me to be attentive to non-verbal cues. For example, I noticed in one session that a resident's head was bent low and his eyes were fixed on the floor. It wasn't until I went to speak with him that he indicated by pointing and shaking his head that he wanted to be taken back to his bedroom. On the day of a sharing, another resident appeared to be pleased when I told her that we were doing a performance. However, it became apparent when we began to set out chairs that she had not understood there would be an audience. She became visibly uncomfortable and it was important that we provided an alternative role for her to have in the day which did not involve performing.

By including these examples, I do not mean to suggest that the difficulties of informed consent were resolved. Rather, I hope to make explicit the ways in which these ethical dilemmas are a central part of the practice.

Relationships of trust developed slowly as residents and I got to know each other and my ability to understand consent developed gradually from being with them, as well as from the ongoing guidance of the people who knew them best. As well as treating consent as an ongoing process, conducting research with people with dementia requires researchers and practitioners to be attuned to the ways that consent may be expressed or withdrawn in conjunction with family and carers, through body language, and through the changing dynamics of the space.

Notes

1. A detailed overview of the Timeslips history and method can be found on the Timeslips website https://www.timeslips.org/, and also in Anne Basting's book *Forget Memory*.
2. This process is documented in the evaluation of their programme RADIQL (Reminiscence Arts and Dementia Impact on Quality of Life), available at https://www.age-exchange.org.uk/what-we-do/inspired-caring/radiql.

References

Arts Council England. (2013). *Arts and Older People in Care Commissioned Grant 2013: Guidance for Applicants*. Retrieved October 20, 2015, from http://www.artscouncil.org.uk/media/uploads/pdf/Arts_and_older_people_in_care_grant_guidance_notes.pdf.

Baring Foundation. (2018). *Each Breath is Valuable—An Evaluation of an Arts in Care Homes Programme*. Retrieved August 6, 2019, from https://baringfoundation.org.uk/resource/each-breath-is-valuable-an-evaluation-of-an-arts-in-care-homes-programme/.

Basting, A., Towey, M., & Rose, E. (2016). *The Penelope Project: An Arts-Based Odyssey to Change Elder Care*. Iowa: University of Iowa Press.

Begault, M., Hodson, K., & Langford, S. (2017). *Magic Me's Artist Residencies in Care Homes*. Retrieved September 1, 2019, from https://magicme.co.uk/wp-content/uploads/2018/03/Artists-Residences-in-Care-Homes-report-WEB-low.pdf.

Department of Health. (2009). Living Well with Dementia: A National Dementia Strategy. Retrieved April 3, 2015, from https://www.gov.uk/government/publications/living-well-with-dementia-a-national-dementia-strategy.

Department of Health. (2012). Prime Minister's Challenge on Dementia. Retrieved April 3, 2015, from https://www.gov.uk/government/uploads/system/uploads/attachment_data/file/215101/dh_133176.pdf.

Goffman, E. (1990). *The Presentation of Self in Everyday Life*. London: Penguin.

Hallam, E., & Ingold, T. (Eds.). (2008). *Creativity and Cultural Improvisation*. London: Berg.

Harris, B. (2013). *The Storybox Project: Examining the role of a theatre and arts-based intervention for people with dementia*. Manchester: The University of Manchester.

Hebdige, D. (1979). *Subculture: The Meaning of Style*. London: Routledge.

Hughes, J., & Nicholson, N. (Eds.). (2016). *Critical Perspectives on Applied Theatre*. Cambridge: Cambridge University Press.

Jackson, S. (2011). *Social Works: Performing Art, Supporting Publics*. Oxon: Routledge.

Jones, C., Tudor Edwards, R., & Windle, R. (2014). Social Return on Investment Analysis of an Art Group for People with Dementia. *The Lancet, 384*, 2.

Keating, F., Cole, L., & Grant, R. (2018). An Evaluation of Group Reminiscence Arts Sessions for People Living with Dementia in Care Homes. *Dementia*. https://doi.org/10.1177/1471301218787655.

Nicholson, N. (2002). The Politics of Trust: Drama Education and the Ethic of Care. *Research in Drama Education, 7*(1), 81–91.

Nicholson, H., Handler, S., Johnson, R., Hatton, N., Lloyd, J., & Sears, R. (2014). Summative Evaluation of Hearts and Minds. A Three Year Pilot Programme by Age Exchange Theatre Trust. Royal Holloway, University of London. Retrieved September 17, 2018, from http://www.eyesociation.org/AgeExchange/SummativeEvaluationHeartsandMinds.pdf.

Schechner, R. (2003). *Performance Theory*. New York: Routledge.

Thompson, J. (2015). Towards an Aesthetics of Care. *Research in Drama Education, 20*(5), 430–441.

Twigg, J., & Martin, M. (2015). The Challenge of Cultural Gerontology. *The Gerontologist, 55*(3), 353–359.

PART I

A Cultural Response

CHAPTER 2

A Cultural Response to Dementia: Moving Beyond the Wellbeing Agenda

Caring Values

> Dementia is one of the biggest global health crises of the 21st century. (Hughes 2017)

It is estimated that there are currently 850,000 people living with a form of dementia in the UK, with Alzheimer's Disease accounting for 62 per cent (see Alzheimer's Society 2019). This figure is expected to double in the next 30 years, rising to 2 million by the year 2051 (Ibid.). The UK's ageing population is the biggest risk factor for this increase as the risk of getting dementia increases with old age. There are now more people of pensionable age in the UK than are under 16. A 2009 report by David Cutler for the Baring Foundation estimated that, in 2003, there were '20 million people aged 50 or over' and that this figure will be '27.2 million by 2031' (Cutler 2009, p. 6). The fastest growing age group of pensioners is 85+, who now make up 4.5 per cent of the population: 'an increase of 45% in a half century' (Ibid.). According to Alzheimer's Research UK, 1 in 3 people who were born in the UK in 2018 will develop dementia in their lifetime (Alzheimer's Research UK 2019).

With no cure and the number of people developing dementia increasing each year, the task of providing high quality, affordable care has become one of the biggest economic, health and social care challenges faced by the Global North in the twenty-first century. The prevalence of people living with dementia in care homes in the UK rose from 56% in

N. Hatton, *Performance and Dementia*,
https://doi.org/10.1007/978-3-030-51077-0_2

2002 to 70% in 2013 (Ibid.). Dementia has been referred to by policy makers as a 'global crisis' (Department of Health 2013), by the neurologist Andrew Lees as a 'silent plague' (2012), and by broadsheet and tabloid newspapers alike as a 'ticking time bomb' (Sheldrick 2015; Furness 2012; Featherstone 2015). The difficulty of providing care and support for an increasing number of people was intensified in the UK by the government's 2015–2020 spending review, which included a £1 billion cut to the social care bill. This placed greater burden on the NHS, and A&E departments in particular, who typically receive a large number of admissions of people with dementia. Statistics published by the BBC in 2015 suggested that over a quarter of hospital beds in England were currently occupied by people with dementia (Gallagher 2015). An inquiry by the Health and Social Care committee at the end of 2016 affirmed that this so called 'bed blocking' was a result of 'delayed transfer of care as a result of not having adequate social care packages in place' (2016, p. 23). Their report also revealed that local authorities, who are responsible for how much they spend on social care suffered a 'real-terms reduction in governmental funding by 40% (Ibid., p. 27) in the last spending review, leading to a massive reduction in the overall availability of social care.

While the number of care home residents with dementia are increasing, the majority of people with dementia are still cared for by family members at home. Writing in *The Guardian* in 2015, George McNamara, head of policy at the Alzheimer's Society, remarked that 'families already shoulder two-thirds of dementia's financial burden through fees and unpaid care' (Featherstone 2015). This means that the majority of dementia care isn't visible and the burden on families goes unnoticed. The implications of the rise in dementia rates and the dismantling of social care provision are particularly bleak for carers of the 'sandwich generation'—those who are simultaneously caring for parents and children. As the average age of first-time parents increases, the financial burden of supporting children and elderly parents means that many are 'struggling to cope financially' (Hughes 2017), as well as increasing the risk of developing health problems themselves.

It is difficult to predict the long-term effects of Brexit on social care policy and practice in the UK. Many, however, have indicated that it will have a substantial effect on the care workforce, a large proportion of which are made up of European migrants. A report by the charity Independent Age in 2018 indicated that 'in the first part of 2016 alone, over 80% of all migrant care workers who moved to England to take on a social care role were from Europe', and that 90 per cent of these migrants do not have British citizenship (Independent Age 2018, p. 2). They raise legitimate concerns that 'if thousands of EEA migrant care workers lose their right to work in England as a result of post Brexit immigration changes, it will be almost impossible to close the already sizable social care workforce gap' (Ibid., p. 27). The implications of these gaps in funding and in staffing, with rising rates of dementia, are likely to have dire consequences for both NHS services and families who are struggling to continue to care for relatives at home.

Underlying this economic crisis is a historical and cultural undervaluing of care as a profession. Care work is low paid, precarious, and often accompanied by low status. It is a workforce which is made up disproportionately by women migrants, many of whom have additional caring responsibilities for family members. Though stories about care in the UK media are typically framed around a care crisis, the issue of sector reform repeatedly fails to gain momentum within the political process. As the journalist Madeline Bunting observes, 'there are few public narratives which describe [caring] attributes, let alone celebrate or affirm them ... In a culture which promotes independence, productivity, achievement, beauty and speed ... the consequences for those who do not meet up to these measures are cruel and we lose sight of the relationships of care on which we are all dependent at some point in our lives' (BBC Radio 3, 2016).

Another factor which has contributed to the crisis status of dementia in the West, and perhaps, to our refusal to address the problem of social care with enough urgency, is the fear and stigma that is associated with a diagnosis. As the playwright and performance scholar Anne Basting identifies, connections between memory and identity are culturally ingrained and contribute to a dominant narrative in which a dementia diagnosis is synonymous with a loss of self. Speaking in the context of North America, she argues that Alzheimer's 'has become something much more than the disease. It has swollen into a fear that permeates the cultural consciousness of the United States ... These fears tap a common source, which is that people with Alzheimer's lose something of enormous value in American culture, their individuality—their "selfhood" (Basting 2003, pp. 88–89). Her view is one shared by the British arts and ageing researcher Hannah Zeilig, who argues that under the conditions of late capitalism, dementia has become a 'cultural metaphor' for tragedy in the Western world (Zeilig 2014, p. 258). In considering how dementia is typically represented in the

British media, she observes that it has ominously been described in meteorological terms, as a 'silent tsunami', 'a rising tide', and a 'galactic storm' (Ibid., p. 260). Basting and Zeilig's observations on the stories that are told about dementia point to the way in which it is perceived as a loss of identity on an individual level, but also as a societal epidemic of biblical proportions. Their research indicates that, in addition to being a set of neurological symptoms, dementia is also a socially constructed phenomenon which is exacerbated by our cultural fears about memory loss.

Despite the fear and stigma that is associated with dementia, Basting suggests that understanding how memories are constructed culturally and relationally can challenge the idea that a person's memory is constitutive of their identity:

> Like identity, which is always personal and social, memory can never be a solely individual act. Memories are formed within culture and triggered through culture. Memory, therefore, can be used to affirm and define self, but always in relation to others. This is the hubris that Alzheimer's narratives expose: we cling to the notion that personal memory alone constitutes selfhood. (Basting 2003, p. 97)

Basting suggests that the 'narrative' of Alzheimer's Disease can be understood in different ways and that the personal experiences of those living with dementia can contest these deep-rooted connections that exist between memory and self. This assertion is strengthened through her creative practice with people who are living with dementia. Writing about a creative writing programme that she led in a residential care facility, she describes a participant called Cary who kept a journal about his experiences of living with dementia. She observes how Cary expressed, in a fragmented fashion, 'longings for his former life, dread of stairs, passion for music and history, fondness for his little dog, hunger for knowledge, bouts of loneliness and confusion, and empathy for his caregiver' (Ibid., p. 94). Cary's journal was significant because it revealed a narrative voice that 'lived in the present moment' and 'did not rely heavily on memory to define who he was' (Ibid.). It also illustrated that there were more ways for people with dementia to express their identity than simply 'parading one's control of memory' (Ibid., p. 97). The journal entries that she describes show how Cary's identity was defined through a number of different but interrelated factors, including his personal qualities, his relationships with significant others, his hobbies and interests, and his emotional responses to his condition.

Basting's ideas on the cultural construction of memory raises questions as to how those engaged in cultural practices respond to the dementia care crisis. In the same way that she has used the stories of people with dementia to challenge individualised concepts of selfhood, concepts which rely heavily on a person's capacity to remember, this book argues that arts practices in care homes can support a concept of selfhood in dementia which is based on interdependence and relationality. By investigating how people with dementia express and negotiate their identities in relation to the creative work, to each other, and to the wider care home community, its aim is to explore how artists can support dementia care as a relational practice. By investigating the intersection between participatory arts and the creative life of a care community, it argues that dementia care should be regarded as a creative practice in its own right.

The Problem with Wellbeing

In understanding the need for a cultural response to dementia, it is necessary to examine how the field of arts and dementia developed in the UK in response to particular strategies in the health sector. Policies such as the *National Dementia Strategy* (2009) and *The Prime Minister's Challenge on Dementia* (2012) attempted to shift public thinking away from an attitude that 'nothing can be done' for people with dementia (Department of Health 2012, p. 3), and to look at strategies for improving their quality of life. This focus on quality of life led to greater primacy being placed on non-clinical interventions, including a therapeutic interest in how the arts can support wellbeing. Until recently, the majority of research that has taken place about the arts in dementia care has focused on its potential to improve the wellbeing of participants. A report written by The Baring Foundation in 2011, for example, explored 'how the arts can contribute to wellbeing and quality of life in residential care' (Cutler et al. 2011, p. 1). This research was matched by a body of academic evidence which assessed the health benefits of participation.[1] As the theatre scholar Caoimhe McAvinchey remarked in her investigation of arts practices with older people, 'there is now a growing body of research that provides compelling evidence about the impact of participation in the arts on people's well-being' (McAvinchey 2013, p. 361).

While this research is important in understanding the health benefits that can come with participation, it only offers one perspective on the value of the work. Furthermore, the status of wellbeing within public policy in the UK risks limiting the scope of enquiry about the value of the arts in dementia care. As McAvinchey suggests, 'if we only ask questions about the social, economic and health value of the arts with older people, we continue to develop an evidence base that reiterates particular, already known, outcomes' (Ibid., p. 361). An additional problem with this type of research is that the concept of wellbeing can be problematic for people with dementia, who may not conform to the criteria that is required for achieving it. In the following section, I outline how a 'wellbeing agenda' emerged in the UK and why I think it is a problematic concept for people with dementia. I then explain how this agenda has influenced arts practices in dementia care, and why a cultural response is needed.

After the Conservative-led coalition government formed in 2010, the concept of wellbeing became a key policy area for the then Prime Minister David Cameron. In a speech delivered that year, Cameron launched a National Wellbeing Programme, with the aim of 'measuring our progress as a country' and understanding 'how our lives are improving; not just by our standard of living, but by our quality of life' (Cabinet Office 2010). Since then, the Office of National Statistics (ONS) have developed several strategies for measuring the nation's wellbeing, including a National Wellbeing Survey, and a series of publications that are designed to capture different aspects of public wellbeing (see ONS 2011, and www.ons.gov.uk).

The National Wellbeing Programme made wellbeing a prominent concept within the public imagination. However, defining what wellbeing is can be a difficult task. The ONS acknowledge that wellbeing 'is a broad term which covers a range of things' (ONS 2011, p. 6), but attempt to define it as follows:

> well-being includes both subjective and objective measures. It includes feelings of happiness and other aspects of subjective wellbeing, such as feeling that one's activities are worthwhile, or being satisfied with family relationships. It also includes aspects of wellbeing that can be measured by more objective approaches, such as life expectancy and educational achievements. (Ibid., p. 2)

The theme of work and family relationships was reiterated in Cameron's speech, in which he stated that the wellbeing policy was connected to 'our goal of trying to create a more family-friendly country ... I want every decision to be judged on whether it makes our country more or less family friendly and this new focus on well-being I believe will be an important part of that' (Cabinet Office 2010). He went on to suggest that '...having the purpose of a job is as important to the soul as it is to the bank balances' (Ibid.). This sentiment was echoed in former Prime Minister Theresa May's 2017 article on the Shared Society. In it, she emphasised the link between the wellbeing of employees and productivity in the workplace: '...mental wellbeing doesn't just improve the health of employees, it improves their motivation, reduces their absence and drives better productivity too' (*Sunday Telegraph*, 2017).

The concept of individualised wellbeing has been praised by some, such as the political commentator Pat Kane who believes that it extends economic concepts of wellbeing and represented a 'much-needed gentler response to the economic crisis' (Kane 2011). However, the political writer William Davies, and others, have expressed a 'growing unease with individualised concepts of wellbeing and the way in which notions of happiness and wellbeing have been adopted by policy makers' (Davies 2015, p. vi). He believes that there is a risk that 'science ends up blaming—and medicating—individuals for their own misery and ignores the context that has contributed to it' (Ibid.). The All-Party Parliamentary Group on Arts, Health and Wellbeing acknowledge the 'pitfalls of individualism' (APPGAHW 2017, p. 19) when looking at wellbeing in an arts and health context. These pitfalls are particularly apparent if we consider the assumptions that wellbeing rhetoric makes about capacity and social networks.

The emphasis that David Cameron's speech placed on family life as a fundamental aspect of wellbeing is problematic for those who live in care homes, who no longer live with family and may have lost their support network in the transition to residential care. Similarly, the idea that employment provides a sense of purpose may mean little to people with dementia who are no longer working and are unlikely to ever do so again. This issue is taken up more broadly by the sociologists Claire Edwards and Rob Imrie, who consider the particular implications of the wellbeing agenda for people with disabilities. They criticise the 'implicit assumptions' that they believe are embodied in the policy, namely that 'life satisfaction is related to particular idealised forms of behaviour or ways of being (including being healthy, fit, employed and engaged in civil society) which engender positive emotional states' (Edwards and Imrie 2008, p. 338). Their criticisms of the wellbeing agenda are pertinent to those living with dementia, who may never be able to contribute to the economy or conform to this idealised version of citizenship. This problem is highlighted further by a lack of representation of people with dementia from the National Wellbeing Survey. Although the Office of National Statistics claims to have consulted a cross-sector of the British public including 'retired people' (ONS 2011, p. 5), there is a conspicuous absence of responses from people living with dementia or those living in care homes. Additionally, though the report claims to have consulted 'disability groups' (Ibid.), there is no specific information about the responses from these individuals, or what type of disability they are referring to.

At the centre of Edwards and Imrie's criticism of the wellbeing agenda is the responsibility that has been placed on the individual in achieving or maintaining their own wellbeing. Drawing on analyses from the sociologists Frank Furedi and Nikolas Rose, they suggest that the wellbeing agenda is symptomatic of a 'politics of happiness', in which governments are 'increasingly concerned with the management of individual emotions and behaviour, as a consequence of a growing tendency to redefine public issues as the private problem of the individual (Edwards and Imrie 2008, p. 338). This idea is shared by the sociologist Eeva Sointu who suggests that in a consumerist society such as the UK, wellbeing emerges as a 'normative obligation chosen and sought after by individual agents' (Sointu 2006, p. 55). Such an approach to wellbeing, they argue, overlooks the 'significant societal barriers that particular individuals, such as those with disabilities, experience in participating in society as self-determining citizens and, through a reductive analysis of emotions, further stigmatise those who do not meet the wellbeing ideal' (Edwards and Imrie 2008, p. 338). When seen in this light, there is a risk that that artists working in dementia care settings may collude unintentionally with an agenda in which responsibility is placed with the individual for maintaining their own wellbeing. This is not to say that artists who work in care homes should avoid therapeutic outcomes, but that the pressure to demonstrate improvements in wellbeing may contribute to a neoliberal agenda, in which the welfare of people with dementia is situated as an individual's 'problem', rather than as something which is the responsibility of health and social care services.

In her book *Fair Play*, the theatre scholar Jen Harvie suggests that there is a need to consider how participatory art and performance practices 'might productively resist but also, damagingly contribute to neoliberal governmentality' (Harvie 2013, p. 16). Harvie is writing about a different type of participatory art, the type which invites dialogic exchange rather than the type where participants are co-creators of the work, such as in an applied or community setting. However, her observation is pertinent to artists who are working in dementia care settings, for whom providing quantifiable evidence about improvements in wellbeing can be a necessary part of securing funding and ensuring the continuation of the work. This is particularly true if the work is funded by organisations for whom cost effectiveness and measurable health outcomes are prioritised.

The cultural policy researchers Eleonora Belfiore and Oliver Bennett outline some of the broader limitations of evidence-based research when it is used to assess the impact of the arts on society or a particular group. In *The Social Impact of the Arts*, they describe how the notion of transformation has historically dominated policy debate about the value of the arts in the UK. They argue that, in an era of financial austerity, claims about the capacity of the arts 'to transform the lives not just of individuals but of whole communities' (Belfiore and Bennett 2008, p. 2) have become a familiar refrain in the case for state funding. This mean that the arts 'occupy a fragile position in public policy', because the claims that are made for transformation 'are extremely hard to substantiate' (Ibid., p. 5). Belfiore and Bennett suggest that this fragile position has been exacerbated by the 'growing prominence of evidence-based policy making', which is widely perceived to be the 'gold standard' of research in public policy (Ibid.), and an economic desire to understand the effectiveness of the arts in achieving pre-determined outcomes.

One of the particular difficulties of attempting to measure wellbeing in an arts and dementia context is that, in addition to being a very difficult thing to define, wellbeing is a subjective experience that does not easily fit within the framework of a scoring mechanism. As the sociologist Bethan Harries outlines in her evaluation of STORYBOX, a drama-based storytelling programme for people with dementia, the use of scoring mechanisms suggests 'a simplification of well-being and infers each measure is uniformly experienced' (Harris 2013, p. 9). In theatre and performance work, attempts to measure the impact that a project has had on participants with scoring mechanisms pose further difficulties because they do not necessarily 'fit' with a performance process. This issue is taken up by the arts therapist Andrea Gilroy in her investigation into evidence-based research in arts therapy. She suggests that 'outcomes are particularly problematic when the 'treatment' being evaluated cannot be broken down into measurable component parts' (Gilroy 2006, p. 10).

The issues raised by Gilroy, Harries, Belfiore and Bennett demonstrate the limitations of arts and dementia research which focuses exclusively on wellbeing, or which relies solely on quantitative measures to interpret the value of the work. Furthermore, the task of measuring wellbeing, which in quantitative research often requires participants to reflect on how they felt before and after a workshop, is made even more problematic in dementia care settings because participants may communicate non-verbally or may not remember taking part. These issues indicate the need to broaden the scope of inquiry, but also to explore what arts-based research methods might offer in understanding the wider value of the work. In an evaluation report for *RADIQL*, a Reminiscence Arts programme for people living with dementia, the research team argue that that 'research methods drawn from the arts provide a context for the quantitative study by critically engaging with the 'how' and 'why'; a process of questioning that clarifies and defines the specific artistic, aesthetic and communitarian qualities of Reminiscence Arts' (Nicholson et al. 2015, p. 6). Their perspective is useful in understanding the methodological importance of arts-led research in this context.

A 2018 evaluation of the Arts Council's *Arts in Care Homes* programme, written by the Baring Foundation, indicated a shift in emphasis from wellbeing outcomes to building a 'body of arts knowledge' (Baring Foundation 2018, p. 45) which centres on 'value of collaboration between the arts and care sectors' (Ibid., p. 4). The report attended to the how and the why of the partnership by looking at 'high quality creative practice', 'challenges in partnership and 'the value of a more embedded cross-sectoral approach' (Ibid., p. 5). This book builds on these creative and collaborative concerns by considering how artists and arts-based research can attend to the wider social, environmental and cultural conditions in which caregiving takes place. By situating creative practice in relation to the everyday routines of a care home, it explores how and why the arts can support dementia care as a relational practice. Drawing a parallel between participatory arts practice and the everyday creativity of a care home, it considers what the aesthetic and social qualities of arts practices can offer in supporting the care home as a creative place.

Theoretical developments in critical disability studies are also valuable in understanding the contribution that the arts can offer to our cultural understanding of dementia. The disability researchers Dan Goodley and Katherine Runswick-Cole propose an alternative to individualised concepts of selfhood in disability studies with their theory of 'dis/human studies'. Dis/humanism considers how people with intellectual disabilities contribute to alternative understandings of humanity and citizenship. Expanding on Rosi Braidotti's concept of the post-human, they use the term 'dis/human' to interrogate the 'ambivalent relationship that disabled people with intellectual disabilities have towards traditional notions of the human' (Goodley and Runswick-Cole 2014, p. 3). Their intention is not to reject the idea of the human outright but to question, as Edwards and Imrie do, the kinds of humans that are currently valued by society. By exploring humanism through the lens of disability, their aim is to explore how disability 'enlarges, disrupts, pauses, questions and clarifies what it means to be human' (Ibid., p. 2).

What is particularly relevant about their concept of dis/humanism is its emphasis on 'interdependence, mutuality and interconnection' (Ibid.). Their theory challenges humanist concepts of selfhood by suggesting that self is always defined in relation to others. Dis/humanism recognises the 'relational rather than the individual nature of autonomy in the lives of disabled and non-disabled people' (Ibid., p. 10). Evoking Giles Deleuze's image of the assemblage, they argue that thinking about the self as an interdependent rather than an individualised being supports the idea of a 'distributed competence', in which a person with disabilities is advocated by a network of interdependent relationships.

In order to explain what this network might look like, Goodley and Runswick-Cole describe a model of community living called Circles of Support. A Circle of Support is a group of people that a person with learning disabilities choose to support them in different areas of their lives. They describe one of the users of Circles of Support, a young man called Matt who has used his disability benefits 'to recruit a network of advocates and support staff to support him 24/7 in his own home' (Ibid., p. 10). This Circle of Support enables Matt to draw on 'myriad forms of community support' (Ibid., p. 11) in order to live independently. They explain that, 'like any good collective, Matt gets lost in the multitude of helping hands and collective gestures … and becomes enveloped within the community assemblage' (Ibid.).

Goodley and Runswick-Cole's description of Matt's 'collective' evokes Basting's argument that self is always expressed in relation to others, and that the identities of people with dementia are constituted by a range of interdependent factors. In the same way that the man in Basting's story revealed an identity which was constituted by a number of significant 'others', such as his dog and his caregiver, dis/humanism raises important questions about how identity might be constructed relationally in a dementia care context.

This book draws a connection between the relationality of participatory arts practice and the relational potential of dementia care. It explores how artists who are working in dementia care settings might use their work to support dementia care as a relational practice. In the following chapter I use the concept of the collective as a starting point for re-thinking dementia care as an interdependent process. Drawing on critical insights from performance studies and human geography, I go on to explore how concepts of atmosphere, sensoriality and affect intersect with this idea. In doing so, I hope to demonstrate how the arts can challenge how we think about dementia, in particular, the idea that a dementia diagnosis is synonymous with a loss of identity.

Creativity and Relationality

Understanding the cultural value of the arts in dementia care is a multifaceted process. It requires arts and health researchers to look beyond individualised notions of wellbeing which have dominated the research agenda until now. By exploring the aesthetic and social qualities of arts practices in care homes, this book begins to address the 'how and the why' that is at the heart of a creative response to dementia care. Focusing on relationship-centred care requires a move away from debates around the instrumental value of the work and to explore what is unique about the arts in promoting caregiving as a reciprocal and creative practice. This move towards relationality not only asks artists to be aware of the wider network of relationships that exist in a dementia care environment. It also requires them to understand the role of the arts in supporting different types of relationality. By exploring the social spaces, atmospheres and sensory exchanges that co-exist in a care home, this book explores how the wider care environment can contribute to the selfhood of people with dementia. Furthermore, it extends current thinking on dementia care by conceiving of caregiving as a creative practice which is shaped by the social, cultural and environmental conditions in which it takes place.

The chapters that follow share stories about the different ways that participatory arts intersect with a care home community. These are stories of creative discovery, of collaboration and of conflict. They recount joyful moments experienced with staff and residents, mistakes and discoveries that occurred at inopportune moments. Crucially, they show how an artists' practice can evolve in response to the network of creative relationships that they are exposed to in a care home. In doing so, I hope that this book will extend current thinking about the arts in dementia care, and about dementia care itself, celebrating them both as relational and improvisatory practices.

Note

1. Key studies include Castora-Binkley et al. (2010) who investigate the impact of the arts on a variety of health outcomes, Camic et al. (2011) who explore the benefits of singing, and 'Dementia and Imagination', an AHRC-funded research project which explores whether the arts can improve the wellbeing of those living with dementia (dementiaandimagination.org.uk n.d.).

References

All-Party Parliamentary Group on Arts Health and Wellbeing. (2017). Creative Health. The Arts for Health and Wellbeing. Retrieved August 8, 2019, from https://www.culturehealthandwellbeing.org.uk/appg-inquiry/.

Alzheimer's Research UK. (2019). Dementia Statistics Hub. Retrieved August 8, 2019, from https://www.dementiastatistics.org/.

Alzheimer's Society. (2019). Dementia UK Report. Retrieved August 8, 2019, from https://www.alzheimers.org.uk/about-us/policy-and-influencing/dementia-uk-report.

Baring Foundation. (2018). Each Breath Is Valuable—An Evaluation of an Arts in Care Homes Programme. Retrieved August 6, 2019, from https://baring-foundation.org.uk/resource/each-breath-is-valuable-an-evaluation-of-an-arts-in-care-homes-programme/.

Basting, A. (2003). Looking Back from Loss: Views of the Self in Alzheimer's Disease. *Journal of Aging Studies, 17*(1), 87–99.

Belfiore, E., & Bennett, O. (2008). *The Social Impact of the Arts: An Intellectual History*. Basingstoke: Palgrave Macmillan.

Bunting, M. (2016). *Crisis of Care* [Radio Essay]. Broadcast on BBC Radio 3, 11 February 2016 at The British Academy. Retrieved August 8, 2019, from https://www.thebritishacademy.ac.uk/events/crisis-care.

Cabinet Office. (2010). *PM Speech on Wellbeing*, 25 November. Retrieved May 29, 2016, from www.gov.uk/government/speeches/pm-speech-on-wellbeing.

Camic, P., Williams, C., & Meeten, F. (2011). Does a 'Singing Together' group improve the quality of life of people with a dementia and their carers? A pilot evaluation study. *Dementia, 12*(2), 157–176.

Castora-Binkley, M., Noelka, L., Prohaska, T., & Satariano W. (2010). Impact of Arts Participation on Health Outcomes for Older Adults. *Journal of Aging, Humanities and the Arts, 4*, 352–367.

Cutler, D. (2009). *Ageing Artfully: Older People and Professional Participatory Arts in the UK*. London: Baring Foundation.
Cutler, D., Kelly, D., & Silver, S. (2011). *Creative Homes: How the Arts Can Contribute to Quality of Life in Residential Care*. Baring Foundation. Retrieved May 28, 2015, from http://baringfoundation.org.uk/wp-content/uploads/2014/09/CreativeCareHomes.pdf.
Davies, W. (2015). *The Happiness Industry. How the Government and Big Businesses Sold Us Well-Being*. London: Verso.
Dementiaandimagination.org.uk. (n.d.). Retrieved July 7, 2020.
Department of Health. (2009). *Living Well with Dementia: A National Dementia Strategy*. Retrieved April 3, 2015, from https://www.gov.uk/government/publications/living-well-with-dementia-a-national-dementia-strategy.
Department of Health. (2012). Prime Minister's Challenge on Dementia. Retrieved April 3, 2015, from https://www.gov.uk/government/uploads/system/uploads/attachment_data/file/215101/dh_133176.pdf.
Department of Health. (2013, December 11). *UK Calls on World to Tackle Global Crisis of Dementia*. Press Release. Retrieved November 30, 2015, from https://www.gov.uk/government/news/uk-calls-on-world-to-tackle-global-crisis-of-dementia.
Edwards, C., & Imrie, R. (2008). Disability and the Implications of the Wellbeing Agenda: Some Reflections from the United Kingdom. *Journal of Social Policy, 37*(3), 337–355.
Featherstone, E. (2015, June 1). Businesses Ignore the Dementia Timebomb at Their Peril. The Guardian. Retrieved November 30, 2015, from http://www.theguardian.com/sustainable-business/2015/jun/01/businesses-ignore-the-dementia-timebomb-at-their-peril.
Furness, H. (2012, March 7). *Dementia Is 'Next Global Health Time Bomb'. The Telegraph*. Retrieved November 30, 2015, from http://www.telegraph.co.uk/news/health/news/9127801/Dementia-is-next-global-health-time-bomb.html.
Gallagher, J. (2015, August 21). Dementia Levels Are 'Stabilising'. *BBC News*. Retrieved November 30, 2015, from http://www.bbc.co.uk/news/health-34001144.
Gilroy, H. (2006). *Art Therapy, Research & Evidence-Based Practice*. London: SAGE Publications.
Goodley, D., & Runswick-Cole, K. (2014). Becoming Dishuman: Thinking about the Human through Dis/ability. *Discourse: Studies in the Cultural Politics of Education, 37*(1), 1–15.
Harris, B. (2013). *The Storybox Project: Examining the Role of a Theatre and Arts-based Intervention for People with Dementia*. Manchester: The University of Manchester.
Harvie, J. (2013). *Fair Play: Art, Performance and Neoliberalism*. Basingstoke: Palgrave Macmillan.

Health and Social Care Committee. (2016). *Impact of the Spending Review on Health and Social Care*. Parliament UK. Retrieved August 8, 2019, from https://www.parliament.uk/business/committees/committees-a-z/commons-select/health-committee/inquiries/parliament-2015/impact-comprehensive-spending-review-health-social-care-15-16/.

Hughes, J. (2017). *This Is One of the Biggest Global Health Crises of the 21st Century*. World Economic Forum. Retrieved August 8, 2019, from https://www.weforum.org/agenda/2017/09/dementia-trillion-dollar-global-crisis/.

Independent Age. (2018). Brexit and the Future of Migrants in the Social Care Workforce. *Independent Age*. Retrieved August 8, 2019, from https://www.independentage.org/policy-and-research/research-reports/brexit-and-future-of-migrants-social-care-workforce.

Kane, P. (2011, November 13). 'The Wellbeing Agenda Isn't Naval-Gazing, It's Innovation and Survival'. *The Guardian*. Retrieved May 3, 2015, from http://www.theguardian.com/commentisfree/2011/nov/13/wellbeing-agenda-navel-gazing-innovation-survival.

May, T. (2017, January 7). I'm Determined to Build the Shared Society for Everyone. *The Telegraph*. Retrieved August 8, 2019, from https://www.telegraph.co.uk/news/2017/01/07/determined-build-shared-society-everyone/.

McAvinchey, C. (2013). Coming of Age: Arts Practice with Older People in Private and Domestic Spaces. *Research in Drama Education: The Journal of Applied Theatre and Performance, 18*(4), 359–373.

Nicholson, H., Keating, F., Cole, L., & Lloyd, J. (2015). *Reminiscence Arts and Dementia Care, Impact on Quality of Life, 2012–2015*. Royal Holloway, University of London. Retrieved November 30, 2015, from https://www.scie.org.uk/dementia/living-with-dementia/keeping-active/files/RH149-RADIQLinterimReport15.pdf?res=true.

Office for National Statistics. (2011). Measuring What Matters: National Statistician's Reflections on the National Debate on Measuring National Wellbeing. *ONS*. Retrieved August 21, 2015, from http://www.ons.gov.uk/ons/guide-method/user-guidance/well-being/publications/measuring-what-matters%2D%2Dnational-statistician-s-reflections-on-the-national-debate-on-measuring-national-well-being.pdf.

Sheldrick, G. (2015, July 21). Dementia Crisis as £23bn 'Time Bomb' Threatens to Sink the NHS. *Express*. Retrieved November 30, 2015, from http://www.express.co.uk/news/uk/592807/Dementia-crisis-NHS-hospital.

Sointu, E. (2006). The Rise of an Ideal: Tracing Changing Discourse of Wellbeing. *The Sociological Review, 52*(2), 255–277.

Zeilig, H. (2014). Dementia as a Cultural Metaphor. *The Gerontologist, 54*(2), 258–267.

CHAPTER 3

Performative Responses and Dementia-Friendly Theatre

This chapter looks at how theatre-makers are responding to dementia outside care homes. It considers how theatrical portrayals of dementia are shifting from the perspective of carers to the lived experience of dementia as more people with dementia are engaged in theatre-making processes. Examining performances that have been made in collaboration with people with dementia, it considers some of the principles of co-creation and how the involvement of people with dementia is encouraging performance-makers to work innovatively with form, text, narrative and space. Furthermore, it considers the emergence of a dementia-friendly theatre movement and how certain venues are working with people with dementia to make theatre-going a more accessible experience.

In the past decade, there has been an increase in commercially produced plays about dementia in Europe and North America. The theatre scholar Michael Mangan accounts for this increase by the fact that dementia has become more prevalent in the public imagination: 'As we become more aware of our ageing population', he remarks, 'dementia becomes a subject that demands our attention … And over the past few years, theatre has responded' (Mangan 2013, p. 144). In her article about performing with dementia, Julie Henderson provides a useful history of the type of plays that have been produced in North America, many of which are narrated through the experiences of family carers:

> All of these plays present families' complex, multi-dimensional experiences with dementia … and most include autobiographical elements, if not the

N. Hatton, *Performance and Dementia*,
https://doi.org/10.1007/978-3-030-51077-0_3

> author's explicit autobiographical story. These plays, however, all focus strongly on caregiver perspectives, (most are structured as narrated by the caregiver), and therefore the lived experience of dementia 'from the inside' remains unexplored. (Henderson 2019, p. 73)

Similarly, many of the plays produced for the UK stage have been themed around the experiences of carers. These include *Inside Out of Mind* by British playwright Tanya Meyers, which explores life on a hospital dementia ward, and *Visitors* by Barney Norris, which focuses on a family's response to caring for someone with dementia. While still dealing with caregiver responsibility, other productions have attempted to convey the subjective experience of dementia by narrating from the perspective of a character who is living with it. Florian Zeller's *The Father*, which opened at the Tricycle Theatre in 2014 and transferred to the West End, tells the story of Andre, a man with dementia who is cared for by his daughter at home. As his memory diminishes over the course of the play, things start to unravel. Susannah Clapp, who reviewed the play for *The Guardian*, focused on the way in which the play used form and language to make the audience feel Andre's anxiety: 'We see and hear what he sees; sometimes we see and hear it twice. We are never given any certainty or explanation. Confusion, suspicion, dismay, hostility are visited on audience and actor simultaneously' (Clapp 2015).

Clapp's comments point to the opportunity that certain types of theatre present in conveying the subjective experience of dementia. By creating a shared encounter with disorienting sounds, fragmented language, and repeated sequences of action, *The Father* allowed the audience to feel something of Andre's experience as he negotiates an increasingly unfamiliar environment. Plays that unfold from this perspective can, as Henderson suggests, 'intervene in the stereotypical treatment of dementia as a disease, death of self, and social terror, and prompt a re-conceptualising of dementia as a complex, embodied, and relational experience' (Henderson 2019, p. 73). They are however, limited in their ability to convey the experience of dementia authentically if they have not 'involved persons with dementia as part of a formal theatre creation process or been performed by persons with dementia' (Ibid.).

In order to explore some of the ways in which people with dementia can take a central role in a theatre-making process, this chapter explores three examples of performance work in depth. The first, *Autobiographer*, was created by writer and sound artist Melanie Wilson in 2012. Wilson's work involved in-depth research and collaboration with The Alzheimer's Society and people with dementia who attended the Croydon Memory Service. Her intention, after working with these participants, was to create a performance which 'illuminated the experience of dementia from the inside without fictionalizing it' (Wilson in Bayes 2012). The performance text used a range of strategies to do this, including multi-rolling, fragmented speech and repetition in what the theatre scholar Michael Mangan described as 'a poetic portrait of the life and internal world of a woman ... who is suffering from dementia' (Mangan 2013, p. 145).

The second production, *Memory Point(s)* was developed by Winchester-based performance company Platform 4 between 2013 and 2015 and involved an extended period of creative workshopping with people with dementia and their carers. The company set out to explore the aesthetic possibilities of collaborating with people with dementia and their carers and to see 'how they, as artists, could work with the families to make inspiring and genuinely original productions' (Platform 4 2013, p. 5). Through these workshops, the stories and memories of participants were incorporated into a multisensory, promenade performance piece, involving objects, music, costumes, sounds, photographs and storytelling. A priority for the company was how they could capture the experiences of their participants in a performance without changing or tidying up the stories or memories that had been shared.

The third example looks at one theatre venue's approach to collaboration. In 2018 the Leeds Playhouse hosted Every Third Minute—the UK's first theatre and dementia festival which was co-curated by a team of people living with dementia. The festival built on their existing work with people living with dementia and the idea of 'dementia-friendly theatre' as something which could be integrated across all aspects of the theatre-going experience. The festival is significant not just because of its manifestation of the dementia-friendly theatre idea, but because of the different ways that experiences of dementia were prioritised and explored artistically.

What I'm interested in pinning down through these three examples is how dramaturgical approaches which are experiential and fragmented may, in addition to offering a more authentic form of representation, be of value to people with dementia as audience members and performers. Productions that prioritise the performance event and its aesthetic effects may be more appropriate than plays about dementia which rely on dialogue, action and plot. By prioritising the performance event, the conventions of postdramatic theatre may offer a more accessible theatrical form for people with dementia, removing the pressure to link performative episodes into a 'coherent' psychological unfolding of narrative. In her introduction to Hans Lehmann's *Postdramatic Theatre*, theatre scholar Karen Jürs-Munby uses the work of disability-led theatre company Graeae, and their use of 'creatively captioned dialogue' in their shows, as an example of postdramatic performance which effectively combines access with estrangement. 'It's main effects ... are created through an alternative dramaturgy that fully incorporates (rather than adds on) the use of sign language, and audio description into the performance writing—effectively combining both inclusivity/accessibility and gestic defamiliarisation' (Jürs-Munby 2006, pp. 5–6). The potential of an alternative dramaturgy for neurodiverse audiences is echoed by Matt Hargrave in his book *Theatres of Learning Disability*, where he argues that 'the interplay between story and theatrical structure is of surprising importance: where disability is concerned, content estranges form and form defamiliarizes content' (Hargrave 2015, p. 7). The notion of an alternative dramaturgy, therefore, offer a useful starting point for investigating the relationship between access and aesthetics in dementia-friendly theatre.

To illustrate the potential of what Graeae describe as an 'aesthetics of access' in a dementia context, my analysis of *Autobiographer* and *Memory Point(s)* will centre on how the performances 'defamiliarized' their audiences by presenting narratives which had not been 'tidied up' for a neurotypical audience. Looking more deeply at the relationship between access and aesthetics, I then unpack the idea of dementia-friendly theatre in light of the Leeds Playhouse's ongoing work with people living with dementia. Reflecting on the theatre's co-creative approach, I consider some of the effects that involving people with dementia as creative consultants is having on the venue. Examining the layers of access that were intertwined through the *Every Third Minute* festival, I explore how people with dementia can shake up the conventions of theatre-going, re-framing it as an interdependent and vulnerable experience. I begin however, with a discussion of *Autobiographer*, and the ways in which the production used immersive techniques to draw the audience into the world of the central character.

'A Multiplicity of Selves': Melanie Wilson's *Autobiographer*

> In dealing with a profound human experience such as dementia, there are only really questions, and be we scientist or artist, we are all with our different questions only adding to the sum of knowledge and care about the subject. It has never been my experience that biomedical science and art are oppositional, their root is the same one, that of interest in the human experience. We merely have different values for accessing that experience. Neither needs the other to survive, but each is revealed and illuminated brilliantly when either happens to turn their lens upon the other. (Wilson 2012)

In this interview with *What's On Stage*, Melanie Wilson is reflecting on the process of creating *Autobiographer*, a performance which features four actors, a small child and an immersive soundscape in a portrayal of an 80 year old woman who is living with dementia. The production was funded by the Wellcome Trust's public engagement in science programme and as such, it had the intention of increasing public awareness about dementia as well as exploring the artistic possibilities of representing dementia 'from the inside'. Wilson's intention was to create something which enabled the audience to experience the disorientating effects of dementia. She said she wanted the audience to feel that they have, 'for a brief moment, brushed up against a state of being lived out by many thousands of people in this country at this moment, but told in a highly engaging, singular and thought-provoking way' (Bayes 2012).

In the performance, the main character, Flora is played by all four actors who each wear the same costume and portray her at different periods in her life. Lines overlap and repeat as the different Floras talk both to themselves and to the audience about different periods in her life. Through this motif, the production evokes the idea that Flora's identity is constituted by multiple Floras which refer to different periods of time and experiences across her life course. Above the audience hang hundreds of lightbulbs of different sizes and wattages which switch on and off and at different speeds throughout the performance. Mangan describes the effect as being 'like the synapses in a brain' (Mangan 2013, p. 147), highlighting the possibilities of theatrical lighting in representing the neurological processes that cause dementia. The immersive soundscape, composed by Wilson, uses both music and ambient sound such as weather, echoes, piano phrases and vocal whispers, which are combined and build towards a 'disorientating crescendo' (Ibid.) at the climax of the play. By placing the audience in the centre of the space and transmitting the audio inwards, they are invaded with sound from every direction, a technique which serves to immerse and disorientate them as they encounter the multiple selves that make up Flora's identity.

At times, the performance text is made up of halting, fragmented sentences and repeated words which represent Flora's confusion:

> I want ... home.
> I'd like to go home.
> At the other end of the
> Telescope.
> Where I'm also waiting to go home. (Wilson 2012, p. 21)

At other points, the language is fluid, lyrical, and heavy with poetic imagery. These sections draw attention to how Flora's sense of self is made up from stories, images and memories from her past:

> When the bird found her.
> She fell to the ground.
> He opened his beak and she fell.
> He opened his beak and sent beauty into the air.
> Sending out into the air a tintinnabulation of such outrageous beauty
> That the girl fell to the ground horizontal with fear. (Ibid., p. 33)

This passage reflects the poetic character of Flora's speech in *Autobiographer*. Mangan also picks up on the richness of the narrative in which '...the fragmentation of the thoughts of the dementia sufferer becomes a poetic principle in its own right, one which generates its own images and rhythms and thus its own unique meanings' (Mangan 2013, p. 147). His interpretation highlights the possibilities of postdramatic performance in legitimising the speech patterns and communication of people with dementia in the way that they are expressed, drawing attention to what is unique and beautiful instead of what makes sense as part of a conventional narrative structure. Coupled with the immersive soundtrack, the performance follows the score of a sound poem rather than a play, and the audience are invited to feel what Flora feels, rather than attempting to unravel the various strands of her speech as a story. By allowing the atmosphere and production elements of the performance to take precedence,

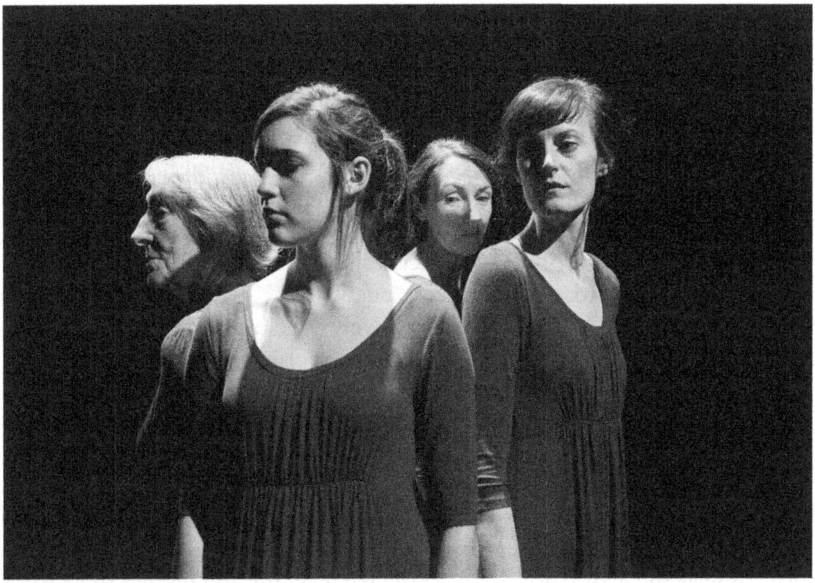

Fig. 3.1 *Autobiographer* by Melanie Wilson. Fuel Theatre. Toynbee Studios, 2011. (Photograph by Monika Chmielarz)

Autobiographer was able to offer a more authentic representation of dementia, one which attended to the fragmentary nature of memories and the sensory experiences of those who are living with it (Fig. 3.1).

While Melanie Wilson's production centred on the internal world of an individual with dementia, Platform 4's production wove together a network of stories that had been gathered from people with dementia and their carers. In *Memory Point(s)*, the fragmented memories of their participants were represented spatially, as well as through sound and images. It was described aptly by Lynn Gardner in *The Guardian* as a 'remarkable collage-style promenade piece' (Ibid.), a description which captures the fragmentary nature of the journey that the audience embark upon as they encounter snapshots in the lives of the participants.

The Aesthetics of Remembering and Forgetting: Platform 4's *Memory Point(s)*

The first phase of Memory Point(s) involved the artists working with people with dementia and family carers over an 18-month period. Participants joined the project through the Southampton and Eastleigh's Connections Club and an Alzheimer's Society service called Singing for the Brain. The timescale of the work marked a radical difference to the 'arts as intervention' approach which often characterises partnerships between artists and people with dementia. This process enabled the artists to get to know participants gradually and to collaboratively develop a form for the performance which they felt best captured the experiences of the participants. The slow duration of the project was captured in an illustrated book which was published in order to document the process as it unfolded. Each chapter moves with the seasons, detailing what the artists learnt as they went along, including their notes, email conversations, photographs, moments of discovery and events, as well as mistakes and wrong turns. This detailed documentation demonstrated the value of allowing the work to develop over time as the artists got to know the participants and gained their trust. It resonated with my own research and practice, and my discovery that artists who are working in care settings need to move towards slower modes of artistic collaboration with people with dementia. This may involve, as the company acknowledge, working with changes and deterioration in memory over the course of the partnership.

The focus of these initial workshops was stimulating the participants' imaginations and memories. The book documents how an early session invited participants to answer the question 'where would you like to go in your dreams?', encouraging them to tell stories about their hopes for the future as well providing opportunities for them to talk about significant places and events from their past. Personal objects were used as a stimulus for evoking memories and the participants were asked to bring in objects that were meaningful to them. As one of the artists explains: 'I wanted to begin the creative process from the perspective of found objects. What memories did these objects conceal? What stories could they tell?' (Platform 4 2013, p. 50). In the workshops, personal objects were discussed as things that get lost and found, and this led to a creative focus on how objects are both lost and accumulated through life. Some participants with dementia spoke about their experiences of losing household objects or finding them in the wrong place, and this became a theme in the final performance: 'Lost objects/the wrong objects being in the wrong place/ keys in oven/kettles in handbags/losing and finding things from your life/dropping and picking things up on the way' (Ibid., p. 36).

The process of accumulating, finding and losing objects was also captured physically in the final performance where personal objects were found in unexpected places. The company explain that the participants' memories are presented as 'pictures, objects, sequences of film, snatches of sound. But they are, above all, fragments; tenderly evoked, they are also left unexplained' (Ibid., p. 9). Towards the end of the performance, the audience is invited to examine a series of tiny and beautifully curated lockers. Each locker contains miniature sculptures, beautifully lit, which depict a snapshot of a particular memory. To access them, each audience member chooses a small key with a number on it and unlocks the locker with the number which corresponds to it. This process draws attention to the privileged position we are given as audience members in glimpsing the personal memories of the participants through these carefully curated stories. As Gardner remarked, 'I have never met any of the couples from Southampton and Eastleigh's Connections Club and Singing for the Brain groups … but I feel that I know them as a result of this show' (Gardner 2013).

I was a participant of the Southbank performance of *Memory Point(s)* in 2014. Rather than being performed in one of the Southbank's designated performance spaces, the performance took place in the basement of the building, an area that is usually off-limits to the general public. The audience, who are guided around the space by actors as well as audio instructions on headsets, are led around the long, dark corridors and dusty corners, backstage areas, cupboards and cubby holes of the building, some of which you feel haven't been visited in years. Like Wilson, Platform 4 attempted to create something of the experience of living with dementia by de-familiarising their audience and taking them out of their comfort zone. The result is disorientating. We are guided through dark corridors. Our attention is directed to particular things by torch light or by an actor's gesture: a ghostly violin player, a day at the seaside, a holiday in the sun. With the immersive soundscape and the continuous twists and turns, I feel a slight motion-sickness, as if I am in the bowels of the ship. The voices of the participants also feature on the audio soundtrack, accompanied by music and sound effects. The company explain their decision to present the participants' memories in the way that they were originally told, including fragments and repetitions: 'No attempt has been made to weld them into a conventional clear narrative, no writer has been hired to draw out the meaning for us' (Platform 4 2013, p. 8). The result of these recorded memories been played through headsets is that we feel as if we have been placed temporarily in the mind of the participants, that we are re-living their personal memories as we follow the winding paths of the performance space.

The journey, which lasts about an hour, includes a series of wrong turns and encounters with seemingly unremarkable places. This 'deliberately disorientating' (Ibid., p. 84) route invites the audience to engage with the mundane. Each nook, corner and corridor is carefully curated to represent a different fragment of memory or time. The company describe how the memories of the participants are deliberately represented spatially: 'memories are tucked away in the places that an audience doesn't usually get to see, the sprawling corridors and awkward spaces, underneath, above and behind that stage. We sometimes feel, as we wander around those dusty, awkward spaces, that we are visiting some kind of museum' (Ibid., p. 48). They explain that this process was a way of encouraging audiences to engage with their immediate surroundings:

> Long intervals of simply wandering about encourage us to reflect on what we are experiencing. The experience may seem like an obscure and shadowy one, until we realise that the curators are shining a light on an experience more fundamental by far: what it might be like to become disorientated, confused and unable to recall. ... It places us in the position of those who are trying to remember. (Ibid., p. 9)

In other words, the journey we are taking is less about the destination and more about walking in the shoes of the participants who have inspired it.

As well as issuing instructions, the headsets play an immersive soundscape which pave our journey around the performance route. Fragments of music, voices and sound fade in and out through my headset. Unsure of which direction to turn, I become reliant on my senses to show me the way. I feel physically lost, out of my comfort zone, but after a while I stop seeking a logical route with which to make sense of my journey. I go with the flow and to start to enjoy each bit of the installation in the moment. Our journey ends on the stage of theatre and we enter from each side of the wings. Just before, we are invited to put on costumes in the dressing room. The costumes relate, in some way, to the memories that we have glimpsed during our journey. A straw hat that was lost on holiday, a sequinned dress from an evening out dancing. A stage manager says each of our names over an intercom and announces our five-minute call. We feel awkward and a bit giggly as we look at each other with a sense of expectation and compliment each other on our costumes. Soon, we are led out from the wings onto the stage to join a group of actors and musicians who are singing, dancing and playing instruments. The lights are hot and bright. Tea and cake is served at tables. There is a party atmosphere but I feel quite exposed, dressed up, standing centre stage and posing for a photograph with my fellow participants. My awkwardness increases when I am encouraged to join hands and dance with another person. There is something a bit odd about being paraded to an empty auditorium. I feel vulnerable and I realise, that this is because I don't know what is coming next. As I look out onto the empty seats in the theatre I am blinded by the lights. I have a thought that the sensation I am experiencing might be similar to that experienced by someone with dementia attending a party at a care home. They may know it is a party because of the atmosphere in the room or the way that the space is decorated. However, they may not necessarily understand where they are or why they are there. I also feel a sense of responsibility in bearing a fragment of someone else's personal memory. There was nothing passive about my journey through the participants' stories, and I left the performance feeling as if I had witnessed something quite fragile and personal. The production highlighted the responsibility that artists have when presenting the memories of others, while simultaneously suggesting to the audience that the processes of remembering and forgetting are intimately entwined.

Memory Point(s) is an example of how involving people with dementia in a performance-making process can inspire innovations in scale, form and temporality. Working with participants from Southampton and Eastleigh's Connections Club encouraged Platform 4 to present their stories in a visual and spatial way that did not rely on a linear narrative. These spatial representations of memories and memory loss have implications for performance practice with people who are living with dementia in care homes. They highlight the importance of the material environment and how it is a fundamental part of a workshop experience, alongside theme, form and content. Paying creative attention to unremarkable objects and finding ways of responding to everyday surroundings can help to construct a care home as a creative space, as well as attending to the embodied experiences of participants as they negotiate this environment. Furthermore, the way that

Platform 4 curated the dusty old space they were working in with great care demonstrated how the principles of caregiving can be embedded within a performance. The idea of care as both an aesthetic resource and a source of support is key to the next section of this chapter, which unpacks the idea of dementia-friendly theatre.

Dementia-Friendly Theatre

I can no longer follow story lines and many would feel it was pointless for me to attend a performance … I hadn't followed the plot, but it didn't matter. I enjoyed sharing a wonderful time with the rest of the audience. I enjoyed the laughter, singing of familiar songs but most of all I enjoyed being part of the experience … the wonderful feeling that only being part of an audience can bring (Mitchell in Taylor 2016, p. 5).

In 2014 the Leeds Playhouse, a theatre with a long history of working with older people, became the first venue in the UK to offer a 'dementia-friendly' performance of its production *White Christmas*. Inviting people with dementia to come in as creative consultants, the theatre implemented a number of changes to the performance that had been rehearsed, based on their advice. This included adjustments to lighting, sound and visual effects, re-working sequences of stage action and adding clearer signage to Front of House areas. Feedback from the author and blogger Wendy Mitchell, who lives with young-onset dementia and was part of the audience suggested that, although aspects of the play's narrative had been difficult to follow, the experience created a welcome familiar *feeling*: that of being part of an audience. In this section, I explore how the venue is working with people with dementia to build layers of access into the theatre-going experience, and how this is fostering a new approach to production based on co-creation.

Some context is necessary in order to understand the development of the Playhouse as a dementia-friendly venue. Nicky Taylor, the Playhouse's theatre and dementia research associate, worked for many years at the theatre as their community development manager. She is now conducting research into creativity and co-production based on her experiences of building dementia-friendly performances at the theatre. In an article she explains how the decision to open up a show to an audience with dementia developed gradually[1] through her long-term work with Heydays, a weekly participatory programme for older people. Taylor noticed that some of the participants had started to experience confusion around attending the group, turning up on the wrong day and struggling with their sense of time. She observed that the format of the group was no longer meeting the needs of many of its participants:

> The practical challenges of taking part in a busy, fast-paced project when experiencing disorientation, difficulties with reasoning and communication, proved more difficult. The stigma and shame of dementia meant many people stopped attending *Heydays* altogether, or struggled on, becoming more distanced from their peers, for whom the connotations of this diagnosis were too challenging to address. People with dementia were gradually losing confidence to attend, becoming more and more isolated. (Taylor 2019a, p. 90)

In 2010 she developed some bespoke creative sessions for people with dementia and their partners. These gentle, exploratory workshops were an opportunity to experiment, working closely with participants to understand their needs and developing new ways of working together.

> Working together with sensitive, inquisitive artists and enabling support workers, we discovered effective approaches included using the senses, voice, gesture and humour to connect people, to help them feel safe, valued and able to respond, confident that opinions and imagination carried no rights and wrongs. I saw people reconnect with their bodies, their sense of possibility and their connection with their partners. (Ibid., p. 91)

Encouraged by what she saw and armed with new creative approaches, Taylor organised some opportunities for small groups of participants to see theatre shows. Planning for these visits included in-depth preparation such as themed workshops, pre-show singing sessions and 'detailed communication about the logistics of the visit' (Ibid.). During the performances she observed that 'people with dementia were alert, able to stay focused, to engage with the characters, emotions and visual impact of the show' (Ibid.), and that there was potential to expand on these supported visits. The dementia-friendly performance of *White Christmas* was offered to a whole audience of people living with dementia and their supporters. It was based on the theatre's format of relaxed performances that were originally developed for young audiences with learning difficulties (Taylor pioneered the idea of 'relaxed performances' which has now become a standard practice for many theatre venues in the UK). Despite the venue's experience of preparing theatre for neurodiverse audiences, it was important to Taylor to undertake in-depth consultation in order to ensure that the theatre 'created dementia-friendly performances with integrity rather than making assumptions' (Ibid., p. 92). A team of people living with dementia were invited to come in as consultants. This method where people with dementia were offered the status of 'expert, collaborator, co-creator' (Ibid.) was integral to the future concept and delivery of *Every Third Minute*.

A key role of the consultants was to offer suggestions about creative adaptations to productions that would make them easier to access. Consultants who were living at different stages of dementia were invited to attend a rehearsal or early performance and give feedback. For those at the later stages, who were unable to articulate their response verbally, Taylor made recommendations based on her observation of moments when they were 'deeply engaged or deeply disconnected from the content' or when she read that someone was 'getting a bit restless in their seat or beginning to stand up as if they want to move away (Taylor 2019b)'. The Playhouse's published guide to dementia-friendly performances explains how some sound levels and effects were toned down and lighting and visual effects were softened on the advice of the consultants with dementia who attended rehearsals. For example, during certain musical numbers where there were layers of activity on stage, Taylor worked with the company to 'strip away some of the additional sounds and movements' that might make it difficult for the audience to focus, whilst 'leaving the feel of the number intact' (Taylor 2016, p. 21).

What I'm concerned with articulating here is the ways that we might look at as these adaptations as a way of understanding the opportunities of co-production. I'm interested in the ways that people with dementia can inspire new approaches to theatre-making which don't just make the production more accessible but change the way we think about processes of creative production. Julia Henderson has used the term 'dramaturgy of assistance' to articulate some of the novel dramaturgical approaches that directors in Canada have developed to support the participation of people with dementia as performers. Her concept offers a means of understanding how dementia-friendly adaptations such as those undertaken by Leeds Playhouse, may become aesthetic features which are woven into the creative fabric of productions. Henderson describes it as 'a dramaturgical approach designed to include and support performers with varying degrees of age-related memory loss, including more severe memory loss such as occurs with dementia' (Henderson 2019, p. 76). In the case of the two plays discussed in her article, techniques included structuring the plays to include improvisation on familiar themes, designing characters that can be played by more than one actor, and marking the set with bold graphics so that blocking is easier to remember. Rather than framing these adaptations as an afterthought to the production that has been rehearsed, these scaffolds are built into the creative process in a way that disrupts conventional processes of dramatic composition.

Reflecting on the adaptations that were made for *White Christmas*, Taylor explains how they required full complicity from each member of the creative team from the acting company to the production staff. However, rather than something that was perceived as an add-on to the production that had been rehearsed, the exchange between the actors, director, and the consultants encouraged the actors to re-evaluate their approach and how they communicated the story of the show. Several actors who were interviewed for the Playhouse's dementia-friendly theatre guide spoke of how valuable this experience was for them: 'the opportunity to revaluate what you are doing on stage for a brand-new audience and making the story as clear as we can make it … was a really useful exercise' (Taylor 2016, p. 23). This process is characterised by Taylor as an exchange of gestures.

> That gesture of 'we want you to know what it's like for us' and then the actors receiving that and processing it, translating it to what they do on stage—it's beautiful sometimes. The care with which actors deliver their performances during dementia-friendly shows is really, really beautiful. The changes are often quite subtle but we know why they're there and we know why they're doing it in that way. (Taylor 2019b)

Dementia-friendly performances place neurotypical actors and production companies in a situation where what they know about their audience is thrown into question. This requires them to be vulnerable and open to new ways of working. As *White Christmas* director Nikolai Foster reflected, 'they've challenged me and invited me to think about the production in a way I wouldn't have considered before' (Leeds Playhouse 2017). Making changes part way through a run can be destabilising and may go against the grain of prior training, experience or instinct. Similarly, inviting people with dementia into rehearsals to speak about their access needs asks them to be open about their own vulnerabilities. This type of vulnerability where each party offer their knowledge as a gesture to the other is concurrent with Matt Hargrave's notion of vulnerability as an 'interrupted value' (Hargrave 2017, p. 118) where structural support and assistance become aesthetic resources in a performance. Hargrave's theory is based on his experiences as an audience member for *Intimacy* (2014), a physical theatre work developed and performed by the dancer Michelle Ryan who developed MS part way through her career. Describing the varied and visible ways in which the audience helped Ryan to do things as part of the show, he posits that a shared state of vulnerability between an audience and a disabled performer 'can upset the myth of the autonomous self' (Ibid., p. 115). Involving the audience in intimate acts of care, he argues, can 'interrupt the mechanisms of performance production and create a complex complicity' (Ibid., p. 123). Though the performance context is very different, the exchanges between actor and consultant in the Playhouse's dementia-friendly performances can also be understood as a sort of complicity in which each party is dependent on each other in order for the theatre event to take place. The experience disrupts frames of theatre-going, establishing a line of communication through which the production that has been rehearsed is renegotiated empathetically. As one of the actors, Tamsin Caroll reflected, 'it becomes a real community of give and take' (Caroll in Taylor 2016, p. 23).

Another component of the Playhouse's dementia-friendly performances which embraces this type of vulnerability is the invitation to a local school group to come see the show at the same time. This intergenerational aspect is, in one way, a gesture to the idea that an accessible performance isn't a simplified version of a show for a specific audience, but a shared experience which is unique and aesthetically interesting. Taylor works with the school before the performance to give the students and teachers a context for their visit and to help them understand that they're part of a special experience. She explained that having a mixed audience is an important aspect of the execution of dementia-friendly performances which helps to create a supportive atmosphere.

> We don't only want people with dementia in that audience. We want a generous audience and we want an audience who have absolutely bought into why they are there on that day, knowing they are giving their full support on that day to someone with dementia who might have different needs from them. (Taylor 2019b)

The complicity of a dementia-friendly performance where both audiences are fully committed to why they are there is, I believe, key to understanding what access aesthetics looks like in a dementia context. An environment which, to revisit Jürs-Munby's description, 'fully incorporates (rather than adds on)' access features, emphasises the interconnectedness and collective responsibility that sits between audience members and the theatre venue in creating a performance that more people can enjoy.

During one particular show, the children who attended the performance took on Front-of-House roles, helping to sell ice creams during the interval and tidying up rubbish afterwards. Taylor reflects on the pleasure with which the children took up this position of responsibility and how it also led to some 'really beautiful interactions' between them and the older audience members. Following Hargrave, this activity could be interpreted as an intergenerational act of support which helped everyone to feel at home in the space. Hargrave defines these sorts of moments as 'an openness to affect … in ways we cannot control and that enrich our sense of being alive, in relation to others' (Hargrave 2017, p. 129). This idea is echoed by the performance scholar Sarah Hopfinger in her article about intergenerational performance ecology where she explores how a mixed-age company of performers 'can become responsive … to their entanglements with each other' (Hopfinger 2018, p. 513) through certain methods of devising performance. For Hopfinger, an ecological approach to devising, which prioritises interactions with natural objects and elements, encourages mixed-age performers to attend to each other with extra responsibility and care. Exploring opportunities for intergenerational support shows how a theatre audience can be galvanised to be supportive actors in an experience which interrupts the conventions of theatre-going and demonstrates interdependence as a viable and visible option. The presence of young people was certainly visible within the fabric of the Playhouse's theatre and dementia festival, where 200 members of the youth theatre devised and staged a new performance, inspired by experiences of dementia. The company's decision to make a piece of theatre which offered a 'unique perspective on living well with dementia' (Leeds Playhouse 2017, p. 7) was an example of how younger voices can help to validate their lived experiences. Moreover, having the youth theatre close the festival with their performance sent a strong message about the responsibilities of the younger generation in shaping cultural responses to dementia in the future.

Every Third Minute Festival

The process of creating *Every Third Minute* gives a deeper insight into how the collective identity and caring responsibilities of a theatre audience is radically realised when a venue opens itself up to this type of interruptive process. *Every Third Minute: a festival of theatre of dementia and hope*, represented an opportunity to put the theatre's experiences in working with people with dementia to the forefront of its creative programming. Funded by a Celebrating Age grant from the Arts Council and Baring Foundation, it ran for seven weeks in the spring of 2018 and featured 12 productions, four of which were new commissions. Each production explored the experience of dementia, were made with people with dementia, or created with an audience with dementia in mind. It also featured pop-up performances, subsidised workshops, talks, seminars and training sessions. The idea for the festival was driven in part by Taylor's disappointment in portrayals of dementia on stage and what she perceived to be a 'lack of understanding by theatre makers making shows about dementia, that people with dementia might come and see those shows' (Taylor 2019b). This frustration helped to shape the concept for the festival which was about sharing more hopeful stories from the perspective of those with dementia along with raising awareness that every three minutes, someone develops dementia in the UK. The performances that featured were a departure from the loss-based narratives that have characterised many plays about dementia. As Taylor explains, it was about 'choos[ing] those stories that aren't currently being told and express[ing] dementia in a more balanced way' (Ibid.). The festival built on the creative consultation model that was developed the during dementia-friendly performances and engaged five people with dementia as curators, each with 'different ideas, personalities and experiences' (Ibid.).Taylor explains that there was an 'element of choosing' the people to be in the room; that the curators were invited to take part because she felt they 'had something to say' (Ibid.), and because they were also capable of being part of quite a demanding process. Rather than representing all people with dementia, the curation process was shaped by the experiences and passions of these particular individuals.

The curators were involved in all aspects of the festival, from programming the plays to advising acting companies during rehearsals, designing marketing material, and choosing workshops to run alongside the shows. This was a voluntary role, but they were offered refreshments and travel support as well as free tickets to any of the festival shows, 'invitations to other Playhouse events and celebrations and gifts/presentations at key points in the festival'. Taylor has commented that several of the curators mentioned that they felt proud to be recognised as part of the Playhouse team when members of staff 'knew who we were and greeted us by name' (2019, personal communication).

Every Third Minute's co-creative approach required the whole venue to find a new way of working. Members of staff across different teams were offered dementia awareness training in order to ensure that they could work closely with the consultants in all aspects of festival design. Rather than asking prospective companies and writers to send scripts or a promotional video of their work, the producers designed a new programming process in which artist were invited to send a personalised film to the curators. The film had to communicate in some way, why they made the show, how they involved people living with dementia in their research and processes, and what they hoped to gain by being part of the festival. This process enabled the curators to experience the ideas of the performances in a more creative and accessible way than having to trawl through scripts. Crucially, it also meant that potential partners were required to think through why they wanted to be part of the festival and gave the opportunity for the curators to weed out companies who weren't tuned in to its ethos. Reflecting on the process, Taylor explains that

> It was fascinating because some people put a huge amount of care into it, and some just sent the promo video. What can you do with that when you've said 'we need you to contribute in a bespoke way'? And the curators absolutely loved it because they said 'we thought we were on X-Factor. We were the ones who could say yes or no', and that's very powerful. We didn't steer them. (Taylor 2019b)

This programming process is a critical example of how the Playhouse built access aesthetics into the festival design. As well as inviting proposals in a format that worked best for the curators, it ensured that the stories that were chosen resonated with their diverse experiences. The impact is visible in the themes of many of the productions which avoid loss-based narratives and instead focus on the richness and complexity of personal stories. There was an emphasis on humour and hope with plays that explored, for example, the joy of personal relationships. *Maggie May*, written by Frances Poet was one of the plays commissioned for the festival and explored the continuation of family life alongside dementia. *The Purple List* by Ian Baxter and Libby Pearson gave an insight into the lives of two gay men as they navigated the care system. The input of the consultants was also visible in the type of shows that were programmed which featured poetry, puppetry, music and song as well as dialogue-based performances with a more conventional dramatic structure.

An important event in the festival programme was *This Is Us*, a scratch performance night which offered a platform for artists who were living with dementia. Featuring a range of performers and art forms, it included the first public performance from Our Time, the group that Taylor had been working with, who shared some of the techniques from their sessions. One of the festival curators, a poet, performed a selection of his work and pianist Pete Grogan performed with his daughter, providing musical interludes between each act (Fig. 3.2). It also featured Wendy Mitchell reading extracts from her book and a guest slot from Cognitive Shift, a duo comprised of shadow puppeteer Ali Clough and musician and composer Leo Nolan, who make improvised music and shadow plays based on Nolan's experiences of living with Alzheimer's. *This is Us* was an important manifestation of the 'generous audience' idea as the audience played an active role in the performance. Each member had an opportunity to give feedback to the performers during the event in a supportive, open forum. For each performance, they were asked to write on a piece of paper a word of encouragement for the artist and a suggestion as to what they should do next. This opportunity for interdependence was enabled by the 'scratch' nature of the event which encouraged interactions between audience members and performers and provided an informal setting for the sharing of ideas that might be excerpts, ideas, or works in progress.

In other parts of the festival, people with dementia acted as consultants for shows in rehearsal. A play that received a lot of press attention during the festival was *Still Alice*: a stage adaptation of Lisa Genova's novel by Christine Mary Dunford. The play was written about a year before Julianne Moore's well-known film portrayal of the Harvard university lecturer who developed young-onset dementia in the middle of her career. The play is distinct from the film in several ways: it is episodic in structure with very short scenes. It includes a character called Herself, who is on stage the whole time and represents Alice's inner thoughts. This decision by Dunford enabled the character of Alice to be portrayed with more autonomy than her filmic counterpart. As Taylor observes of the play: 'when she feels that someone is talking over her or patronising her, Herself

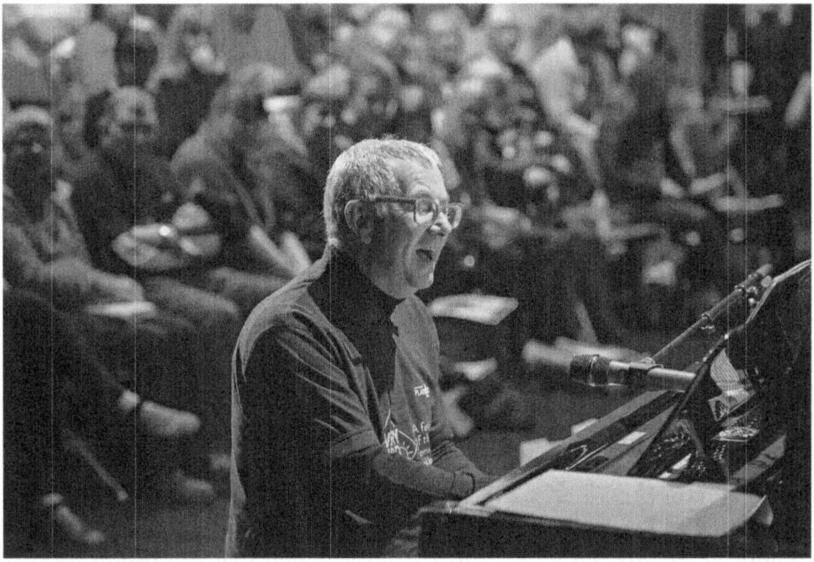

Fig. 3.2 Festival Curator Pete Grogan performing as part of *Every Third Minute Festival*. (Photograph by Anthony Robling for Leeds Playhouse)

articulates that. It's a very clever way of showing that what you're seeing on the outside is only a fraction of what that person's experience is' (Taylor 2019b).

Part of the press interest in *Still Alice* was related to the presence of a known actor, Sharon Small, in the lead role but the angle of many of the articles was how the production team worked with a dementia consultant as part of the rehearsal process (see, for example Yorkshire Post 2018). Wendy Mitchell, the author cited at the beginning of this section was employed as a paid consultant to work with the production team and interviewed by the press alongside Small. As someone who had also experienced young-onset dementia in the middle of her career, her story was not dissimilar to Alice's which gave actor Small a deeper level of access into her character. As Taylor reflects:

> Wendy was an ideal person to be involved as she's completely open and honest and willing to answer really tricky questions that actors want to ask to get under the skin of a character. I was sure that Wendy's involvement would bring the honesty and truthfulness that a production needs. (Ibid.)

Further reflections from the production's director David Grindley provides an insight into some of the specific ways that Mitchell shaped the production process. Mitchell attended the initial read-through and several rehearsals of *Still Alice*, as well as leading a session at the beginning of the rehearsal process with the cast which introduced them to her situation. Grindley explains how Mitchell's openness gave them the confidence to explore the physical as well as the cognitive effects of dementia: 'Wendy was happy for Sharon to copy the effects dementia has on someone's physical capabilities. Sharon was particularly influenced by the care that Wendy has to take when she's walking' (Grindley 2019). This also influenced Grindley's approach to staging. For example, during a scene where Alice gives a lecture about dementia, he used the scene change to show the physical effects of dementia in real time, rather than opting for a smooth transition: 'I decided not to worry about trying to execute it quickly but allow the audience to recognise and witness how Alice walked to the podium' (Ibid.).

As well as teaching the company about the physical considerations of staging dementia, Grindley learnt from Mitchell that the progression of dementia is 'not linear, that some days are better than others, which can perplex those around you' (Ibid.). Mitchell explained that it was:

> ...perfectly possible for her to stand in front of an audience and, with the help of her iPad, give a talk where she would appear to be relatively unaffected by her condition. Yet on other days, she would be unable to leave her chair because it would be too confusing if she did. (Ibid.)

These types of insights can help theatre-makers to present dementia as a complex and individual experience. As well shaping as an actor's interpretation of character, input from consultants living with dementia show how choices about form, structure and staging are equally as important in conveying their stories. In the case of *Still Alice*, Mitchell's involvement enabled some of the nuances of her condition to be translated onto stage and encouraged the company to find creative ways of presenting these details to the audience. Such involvement is necessary if theatre-makers are to avoid making assumptions about dementia and to represent it in a way that is authentic to their lived experiences.

Environmental Adaptations

As with the dementia-friendly performances, the consultation for *Every Third Minute* led to a significant number of adaptations to the venue and the Front-of-House environment, but on a larger scale. A key part of this was understanding how the venue as a whole was experienced differently by people with dementia. 'We did a lot of learning about the venue and how that felt' (Taylor 2019b). The environmental adaptations that resulted included changes to:

> Lighting, signage and visual markers, background music and tannoy announcements to the support offered by our front of house team. We implemented these and also added a quiet space, a relay of the show on a screen in the café for anyone who became unsettled in the auditorium ... flexible seating options and detailed pre-show information to take the stress out of preparing for a visit. (Taylor 2019a, pp. 92–93)

For the purposes of the festival these features were temporary additions. However, their presence over the course of the seven weeks signalled an opportunity for the Playhouse to re-think how their building communicates. Rather than thinking of these features as temporary aids created to support people with dementia during the festival period, these examples indicate how the access requirements of a venue may become permanent design characteristics which signal its openness towards diverse audience experiences. The inclusion of bold, clear signage, flexible seating and quiet spaces may be of value to theatre goers with a range of access needs. This became apparent to me when I attended an *Every Third Minute* performance at a time where I needed extra support.

This time occurred when I visited the festival a few weeks after my first child was born and saw the performance of *Three*—a tryptic of short plays that were co-written by people living with dementia and professional writers. Each performance was 20 minutes long and featured 4 actors who changed roles. While personal memories were a theme that ran through each piece, the stories were very different. The first, *I See Land Ahead* by Bob Fulcher and Dominic Gately was set in a painting class and focused on a long-term friendship told through childhood adventures. The second play, *Hamari Yaadain (Our Memories)* was set in a community memory café for South Asian people in Leeds and featured real-life conversations, woven together by playwright Ming Ho. The third piece, *A Horse Called Freedom* was a dream-like monologue created by Rosa Peterson and Barney Bardsley. It had a more open poetic form and included gentle, live musical accompaniment from a harpist.

During the performance house lights were dimmed in the auditorium but didn't go completely black, which helped to create an informal environment. It also meant that the audience could see each other. The house was not full and there were several rows with just a handful of people in them, providing more space and physical comfort. The set was simple: some wooden stools and carefully placed artists' easels. There were no props and the physical action was distilled, allowing the audience to hone in on the words. On the day I attended I was feeling physically and mentally tender, anxious about leaving my young baby and recovering from a complex birth. By the time I reached the third performance, *A Horse Called Freedom*, I was tired and struggling to focus. Sitting in semi-darkness at the back of the Courtyard Theatre, I stopped trying to concentrate and make meaning from the performance. I put my head back, allowed my eyes to close, and listened to the words and sounds. I didn't feel self-conscious as many other audience members were also accessing and responding to the performance in different ways. Closing my eyes gave me a feel for the rhythm and poetry of the stories and allowed my body to temporarily recover. I felt the vibrations of the harp underneath my feet. I heard someone in the row behind me humming. It struck me that my own access requirements at the time: tiredness, poor concentration, slow mental processing, and the need to dip mentally in and out of the performances, were validated through the caring environment that had been carved out. I didn't bring my baby into the auditorium, but I could quite imagine a situation where I could have done. The flexible environment and supportive atmosphere meant that our circumstances may have been accommodated in a way that they might not have been in other public spaces.

Is a dementia-friendly theatre festival then, an exemplar of an accessible space which can disrupt frames of participation and change the way we think about broader practices of theatre-going? At a time when performance scholars are contesting binary distinctions between performance and participation, might dementia-friendly theatre contribute to an understanding of theatre-going as 'an embodied practice, rather than something that is done to, or by others' (Harpin and Nicholson 2017, p. 3)? Being part of the audience for *Three* certainly opened up a space for me to experience a different mode of theatre-going which was distinct from previously ingrained habits of remembering details, making intellectual connections, and analysing production choices. At *Every Third Minute*, the physical and sensory aspects of the festival experience were 'rehearsed' alongside the productions and were as much a part of the creative process as the performances. This commitment aligns with Harpin and Nicholson's understanding of performance participation as an 'ecology of mutual doings and beings' rather than as 'an invitation and a response' (Ibid., p. 14).

Shortly after the festival, Leeds Playhouse closed for a complete renovation. Taylor suggests that the festival 'informed some conversations' around the design of the new building suggesting that there is potential for some of these access considerations to translate into permanent fixtures. The evaluation for *Every Third Minute* also revealed that the Playhouse are 'investigating how some of our internal processes could be adapted in line with our dementia-friendly approach, which results in greater inclusivity for everyone' (Taylor and Hughes 2019, p. 3). This sort of initiative has the potential to encourage other venues to attend creatively to access. One longer-term effect that is discernible is how the model of collaboration that was developed by the curators at Leeds Playhouse is resonating beyond the festival. A significant creative outcome, identified by Taylor, is that many of the artists involved hadn't worked with people with dementia before but are 'now able to see them as potential collaborators' (Taylor 2019b). The visibility of people with dementia as creative contributors is a necessary step if theatres are to create work which authentically represents their day-to-day lives and experiences. Another important outcome from the festival is that the group are still working together. Since the festival they have given a workshop presentation to the UK Dementia Congress in Brighton and developed creative workshops to deliver with people with dementia in care homes across Leeds. Supporting people with dementia to facilitate creative sessions for other people who are living with dementia is another example of how Henderson's dramaturgy of assistance might work in practice. The participatory scaffolds that are put in place take on a new meaning when framed as an interdependent exchange between people with dementia, who enable each other's participation in diverse ways.

By exploring some of the ways in which theatres and performance makers are moving towards co-creation, this chapter has attempted to make a case for access as an aesthetic choice which supports people with dementia as theatre-goers and theatre-makers. Following Hargrave's notion of vulnerability in performance, it has sought to add a new layer to the debate around disability and aesthetics, analysing some of the specific ways in which dementia productively disrupts processes of dramatic composition. In some cases, the overlap between access and aesthetics has inspired creative approaches which use the experience of dementia to shape the performance event. Favouring poetic language over dialogue, short episodes over long scenes and sensory experiences over unfolding narratives, performances, such as *Autobiographer* and *Memory Point(s)* are examples of how theatre-makers can attend to the shape and feel of dementia.

In addition to embracing new dramaturgical processes, *Every Third Minute* used theatre to increase the visibility of people with dementia, challenging loss-based stereotypes and highlighting the multiple roles that they inhabit. By supporting people with dementia as artists and decision-makers, and representing them in diverse roles on stage, the festival made good on its commitment to offer a festival of theatre, dementia and hope. What the dementia-friendly theatre in this chapter has in common is an emphasis on the embodied knowledge of people with dementia and how this shapes their experiences as audience members and theatre-makers. Identifying participatory scaffolds as aesthetic choices helps us to understand theatre-going as a sensory and relational experience which is enabled through networks of support. This has implications for how theatre practitioners approach their work in care settings, but it also offers an opportunity to think differently about caring relationships. This is the focus of the next chapter, which looks closely at the idea of dementia care through the framework of relationships. Building on the examples of interdependence that can emerge through a theatre-making process, it shows how our approach to care might evolve from an individualised practice to one that embraces (human and non-human) networks of support.

Note

1. For a detailed account of the development of dementia-friendly theatre, see Taylor (2019a) 'The origin of dementia-friendly performances and the role of people with dementia as creative consultants.' RiDE. 24:1, pp. 90–95).

References

Bayes, H. (2012, April 24). *Brief Encounter with … Melanie Wilson*. Retrieved December 15, 2015, from http://www.whatsonstage.com/off-west-end-theatre/news/04-2012/brief-encounter-with-melanie-wilson_4598.html.

Clapp, S. (2015, October 11). The Father Review: Touching Journeys in a Shifting Mindscape. *The Observer*. Retrieved December 9, 2015, from http://www.theguardian.com/stage/2015/oct/11/the-father-review-kenneth-cranham-florian-zeller.

Freeman, S. (2018, February 7). Still Alice: The Play About Dementia Wendy Mitchell Has Helped Bring to Life but Will Never Remember Seeing. *Yorkshire Post*. Retrieved August 19, 2019, from https://www.yorkshirepost.co.uk/news/analysis/still-alice-the-play-about-dementia-wendy-mitchell-has-helped-bring-to-life-but-will-never-remember-seeing-1-9006534.

Gardner, L. (2013). Memory Point(s) review. The Guardian, 2 July. http://www.theguardian.com/stage/2013/jul/02/memory-points-lyn-gardner-review, (accessed 9 December, 2015).

Harpin, A, and Nicholson, N. (2017). Performance and Participation: Practices, Aesthetics, Politics. Basingstoke: Palgrave Macmillan.

Hargrave, M. (2015). *Theatres of Learning Disability: Good Bad or Plain Ugly?* Basingstoke: Palgrave Macmillan.

Hargrave, M. (2017). Dance with a Stranger. Torque Show's 'Intimacy' (2014) and the Experience of Vulnerability in Performance and Spectatorship. In A. O'Grady (Ed.), *Risk, Participation and Performance Practice: Critical Vulnerabilities in a Precarious World*. Basingstoke: Palgrave Macmillan.

Henderson, J. (2019). *Dramaturgy of Assistance*: Performing with Dementia or Age-Related Memory Loss. *Research in Drama Education, 24*(1), 72–89.

Hopfinger, S. (2018). Intergenerational Performance Ecology: A Practice-Based Approach. *Research in Drama Education, 23*(4), 499–516.

Jürs-Munby, K. (2006). Introduction. In H. Lehmann (Ed.), *Postdramatic Theatre*. Oxon: Routledge.

Leeds Playhouse. (2018). Dementia Friendly Performances Information. Retrieved September 1, 2019, from https://www.youtube.com/watch?time_continue=158&v=Fr_7xEkwW00.

Mangan, M. (2013). *Staging Ageing: Theatre, Performance and the Narrative of Decline*. Bristol: Intellect Books.

Platform 4. (2013). *Memory Point(s): The Beauty of Remembering*. Winchester: Platform 4.

Taylor, N. (2016). *West Yorkshire Playhouse's Guide to Dementia Friendly Performances*. Leeds: West Yorkshire Playhouse.

Taylor, N. (2019a). The Origin of Dementia Friendly Theatre Performances and the Role of People Living with Dementia as Creative Consultants. *Research in Drama Education, 24*(1), 90–95.

Taylor, N., & Hughes, V. (2019). Celebrating Age: Every Third Minute Evaluation. Retrieved from www.leedsplayhouse.org.

Wilson, M. (2012). *Autobiographer*. London: Oberon.

Interviews/Correspondence

David Grindley, Director, *Still Alice*. Every Third Minute Festival, Leeds Playhouse, 2018. *Email Correspondence*, 5 June 2019. Ref: Grindley (2019).

Nicky Taylor, Director, *Every Third Minute Festival. Interview*, Leeds 13 February 2019. Ref: Taylor (2019b).

CHAPTER 4

A Relational Approach to Dementia Care

This chapter outlines an approach to dementia care which is inspired by posthumanism. It marks a transition from person-centred dementia care towards a greater emphasis on relationality. Person-centred care was developed by the British gerontologist Tom Kitwood between 1987 and 1998. It was an innovative response to the medical model of dementia care, in which patients were treated chiefly in response to their neurological and psychiatric symptoms. In his most well-known work, *Dementia Reconsidered* (1997), Kitwood argued that this medical model overlooked the social factors which contributed to dementia, and the extent to which some symptoms 'might be due more to failure of understanding and care than to a structural failure of the brain' (3). Kitwood described this medical approach as the 'standard paradigm' (Kitwood 1997, p. 35), and argued that dementia needed to be understood more broadly as an interaction between the personal, the social and the neurological. Consequently, person-centred care takes into account the 'psychosocial' factors that contribute to dementia.

Kitwood's work played a ground-breaking role in the development of dementia care in the UK and abroad. The dementia researchers Clive Baldwin and Andrea Capstick describe him as 'one of the leading figures in the development of our thinking on the nature and process of dementia, the experience of dementia and the development of person-centred care' (Baldwin and Capstick 2007, p. 1). His critique of dementia care culture, his call for a psycho-social understanding, and his proposals for

N. Hatton, *Performance and Dementia*,
https://doi.org/10.1007/978-3-030-51077-0_4

maintaining personhood have been integrated across health and care institutions in the UK and internationally. Training in 'Dementia Care Mapping' and formal qualifications in Dementia Care have emerged from his work, and many care homes use the paradigm of person-centred care to promote their services for the elderly.

Over twenty years later, Kitwood's contribution is starting to be reviewed by dementia researchers in light of theoretical developments in gerontology and dementia studies. One of the criticisms that has emerged from this research is that his concept of personhood is problematic for people with dementia. It is difficult to give a precise definition of this as it is something that he was still articulating prior to his death in 1998. It is also a concept that was influenced by several different disciplines, including theology, social psychology and ethics. As Baldwin and Capstick observe, 'Kitwood was aware of differences in discourses and the 'personhood' they produced … and attempted to combine insights from different discourses into a more complete theory of personhood' (ibid.: 174). There is a recurring philosophical premise that runs through Kitwood's work though, and that is that every person has an ethical status that should be respected and preserved, on account of their '*being* a person' (Kitwood 1997, p. 1, my emphasis). His concept of personhood evolved slightly over the course of his career, but what remained constant was his belief that there was 'an essential unity of human beings' (ibid.: 10), and that this unity was the foundation of a caregiving relationship. 'Rather than emphasize the differences that dementia brings' he argued, 'we will first celebrate our common ground' (ibid.: 8).

For Baldwin and Capstick, this association of personhood with an essential unity is problematic, as it implies humanist values that are necessarily exclusionary. They explain:

> The question 'What is a person?' is an exercise in setting boundaries. By definition there will be those who fall within and those that fall outside the boundaries—that this there are persons and non-persons. The implications that follow from this definitional exercise is that it is permissible to treat non-persons differently. (Baldwin and Capstick 2007, p. 174)

While Kitwood was keen to stress that this unity existed 'whatever differences there may be in mental capabilities as conventionally determined' (Kitwood 1997, p. 10), Baldwin and Capstick suggest that any determination of an essential unity risks excluding those who do not fall within the boundaries of its definition. Dan Goodley considers the problem that such humanist interpretations pose for people with disabilities, or indeed anyone who does not conform to this ideal of personhood:

> Citing the primary signifier of the 'person' evokes with it notions of autonomy and independence: precisely the ableist competencies automatically assumed not to be present in the midst of intellectual disabilities ... in the cold light of day, many of us ... fail to match up to this impossible ideal of personhood. (Goodley 2014, pp. 31–32)

The argument presented in this chapter is that it is relationality, not personhood, which is vital to the caregiving relationship. This is not to say that Kitwood believed that personhood existed independently from relationships. On the contrary, he argued that personhood can only be maintained 'in the context of relationship and social being' (Kitwood 1997, p. 8). This emphasis on relationships was a central part of his theory of person-centred dementia care and later in this chapter I suggest how some of Kitwood's ideas on 'positive person work' (ibid.: 89–93) might support relational dementia care in practice. However, his concept of relationality is underdeveloped. This is partly because it is unidirectional, but it is also because it does not account for the wider network of human and non-human relationships that exist in a caregiving environment. Early conceptions of relationship centred care have rightly positioned dementia care in the context of interdependence. Gerontologist Mike Nolan, for example, has argued for an approach which recognises the reciprocity of caring relationships (Nolan et al. 2004). However, this research does not consider how relationships are formed in dialogue with social, cultural and environmental conditions. As the Canadian dementia researcher Pia Kontos puts it 'even with relationship centred care, the focus remains on care relationships, thus overlooking other relationships that individuals may have such as those with the state and its institutions' (Kontos et al. 2017, p. 183).

My approach expands on existing concepts of relational dementia care by taking into account the wider social and environmental factors which shape the lives of people with dementia, and the context in which caregiving takes place. This context is multi-layered. Not only does it include human relationships, but relationships with non-human artefacts, which share a vital material presence in a care environment. Bringing together ideas on relational care, embodied selfhood and affect, this chapter positions dementia care as an interaction between the human and the non-human. It then explores how the participatory performance techniques, particularly those that are ecologically driven, might nurture these types of caring interactions in practice.

In thinking about dementia care as a posthuman endeavour, I am inspired by the philosopher Bruno Latour's theories on the agency of objects, and his attempt to reconnect the social and natural worlds. In *Pandora's Hope* he contests the humanist logic that society that is made up of subjects and objects, and reconsiders the relationship between humans, natural objects and artefacts in terms of a 'collective' of humans and non-human 'things'. 'Things', as opposed to objects, he argues, are not 'neutral carriers of human will' but are 'entangled' with humans, and share a status of 'actants', in which 'responsibility for action must be shared' (Latour 1999, p. 180). He adopts the linguistic term 'actant', used traditionally to describe the structural roles within a narrative or story, to consider action as a 'property of associated entities and a composition of forces' (ibid.: 182). The political scientist Jane Bennett usefully expands on this definition in her conception of the vitality of matter. 'An actant is a source of action that can be either human or non-human; it is that which has efficacy, can do things … produce effects, alter the course of events' (Bennett 2010, viii). In considering material objects as actants, Latour suggests, we are able to recognise their capacity as 'fully fledged actors in our collective' which have the potential to 'take hold of a passer-by and force them to play a role in its story' (Latour 1999, p. 177). Latour's concept of human and non-human actants is central to this relational approach as it offers a way of thinking about a care home as an interconnected environment of people and things. It can be used to understand the posthuman nature of care spaces and the way in which people with dementia make sense of their environment though sensory encounters.

There are three interrelated components to my approach which are used to position the dementia care in a broader relational context. The first is the notion of relationship-centred care as part of a wider relational aesthetic. In this strand, I develop the interdependent, perceptual, and socio-environmental aspects of relationship-centred care outlined by Mike Nolan and consider dementia care in terms of a network of human and non-human relationships. The second component is the notion of embodied selfhood. Here, I expand on theories of embodied selfhood developed by Pia Kontos and consider how some of Kitwood's ideas on positive person work may be understood in an embodied way. The final component is concerned with the environmental properties of care homes. This is about cultivating an awareness of how sounds, spaces, objects and atmospheres effect the feel of a care home and are key determinants of how they are perceived.

Relationship-Centred Care and Embodied Selfhood

Mike Nolan's concept of relationship-centred care is a useful starting point for understanding the relational potential of dementia care. The overarching principle of his model is that personhood is best understood as a 'network of social relationships ... which are deeply connected and interdependent' (Nolan et al. 2004, p. 47). Though acknowledging the significance of the individual, relationship-centred care focuses on the interdependent nature of care relationships, framing it as a reciprocal and continual process of exchange between the carer and the person with dementia. Using a broader healthcare context to outline the reciprocal qualities of a caregiving relationship, the healthcare researchers Mary Beach and Thomas Inui challenge the 'detached concern and neutrality' that is traditionally associated with a doctor-patient relationship, and suggest that emotion and affect should not only be acknowledged but understood as vital components in developing and maintaining a high quality care relationship (Beach and Inui 2006, p. 3). Their emphasis on the role of emotion, and Nolan's attention to the 'subjective and perceptual aspects' of caregiving, highlight the role of feeling and perception within relationship-centred dementia care, and the interplay between the two, suggesting that each caring relationship is perceived differently and necessarily involves a process of 'getting a feel' for each other.

Nolan expands on the sensing and feeling qualities of relationship-centred care in his concept of the 'Senses Framework'—a set of feelings that a person with dementia and their carer must have 'a sense of' in order to achieve a high quality caring relationship (2004 and 2006). While these six concepts are significant, particularly in offering one of the first conceptual alternatives to Kitwood's 'Flower',[1] it is the perceptual and sensory qualities of his Senses Framework, and the emphasis on 'getting a sense of [something]' that I take forward in my approach.

Nolan argues that in achieving relationship-centred care, 'there is a need to create a 'milieu' in which all participants are meaningfully involved, and which reflects the existence of multiple environments of care' (Nolan 2006, p. 47). Significantly, his suggestion alludes to the role of the environment in dementia care. While relationship-centred care acknowledges that caregiving is made up of a network of different relationships, the term 'relationship' has traditionally referred to relationships between people. This is consistent with Kitwood's concept of person-centred care, which although pays some attention to organisational culture, is generally interpreted as a relationship between two people: the person with dementia and their carer. This is apparent in the way that Kitwood adopts the philosopher Martin Buber's concept of 'I-thou' in order to describe how people with dementia and their carers pay each other mutual respect and attention (Kitwood 1997, p. 10). Nolan's description of the care 'milieu' provokes questions about how the caregiving environment functions as an active component in the caregiving relationship. The notion of a care milieu supports the idea of a care 'collective' by pointing towards the broader network of relationships that exist within a single care home, which is multi-layered, and not only includes relationships between people with dementia, care staff, residents and family members, but relationships with non-human artefacts.

Theories about dementia and the embodied selfoffer some insight into how this 'milieu' might work in practice. Kitwood did, in his original conception of personhood, suggest that his theory might be interpreted in a more embodied way (ibid.: 16). However, as Bartlett and O'Connor observe, this was chiefly suggested in relation to the neurological features of the body, or a 'duality of mind and body', rather than an understanding of corporeal intentionality (Bartlett and O'Connor 2010, p. 183). Drawing on Kontos's work, they suggest that a non-representational theory of embodiment or 'embodied selfhood' may offer insights into how the 'pre-reflective or taken for granted body, as it is engaged in the usual habits and practices of daily life', may tell us more about the experience of living with dementia (ibid.). The concept of embodied selfhood is fundamental to a relational approach in understanding how relationships are negotiated by the pre-reflective body in dementia care, and how people with dementia contribute to caregiving relationships at an embodied level. It is also important in understanding the sensory relationships that people with dementia have with the caregiving environment, how the body attunes and responds to its surroundings, and the information that it receives and transmits through being in the space.

Kontos argues that personhood in dementia care should be understood in the context of the pre-reflective body, where: 'the body is a fundamental source of selfhood that does not derive its agency from a cognitive form of knowledge' (Kontos 2005, p. 555). Theorising the 'agential role' of the body in the constitution of personhood, she draws on phenomenological interpretations of the body as a primary site of knowing. She suggests that existing concepts of personhood in dementia care fail to recognise the significance of the lived body, or at best, relegate it to a symbolic role 'where it is understood as being representative of meaning rather than a significant dimension of selfhood' (ibid.: 553). Kontos' rejection of representationalist interpretations of the body challenges the 'loss of self' narrative which is commonly associated with a dementia diagnosis. For performance practitioners working in care homes, there is an opportunity to consider the material significance of the body, and what it contributes to the care milieu by virtue of its 'being in the world' (ibid.: 563). Furthermore, her awareness of the agency of the pre-reflective body validates non-cognitive forms of communication within dementia care and draws attention to the importance of the lived body as a means of making sense of a care environment.

Baldwin and Capstick acknowledge the importance of environment in embodied selfhood, arguing that embodiment can only be understood as 'situated ... in a social or cultural world that not only provides the sources of these bodily practices but also serve as the background against which they make sense and are meaningful' (Baldwin and Capstick 2007, p. 183). Moreover, Kontos suggests there is a fundamental relationship between a person with dementia's 'pre reflective sense' and their 'grasp of their environment', as evidenced by 'their capacity to move around in and to utilise space without first having to think how to do so' (Kontos 2004, p. 839). Their observations speak to the affective interplay that exists between the embodied self and the care home environment, and the role that the body has in attuning or responding to it. The body's intuitive behaviour or 'know-how', its meaningful habits and gestures, and the sensory interactions that occur in the moment, validate the improvisatory nature of everyday life in a care home and the way that information is absorbed through sensory encounters with the space. Embodied selfhood supports the notion of a dementia care collective, which is made so because of the shared materiality of humans and non-humans, rather than socio-interactive conditions. Furthermore, it supports the concept of relational care beyond cognitive human interactions by drawing attention to pre-reflective, sensory relationships that exist intrinsically between the human body and the non-human properties of the space.

In order to understand how embodied selfhood might be supported in practice, I have revisited some of Kitwood's ideas on person-centred care.

Although Kitwood's concept of personhood has limitations for people with dementia, some of his ideas on 'positive person work' are instructive in understanding how people with dementia express their identity and maintain relationships on a pre-reflective level. There are two particular ideas that Kitwood developed which support the notion of embodied selfhood, and embrace the reciprocity of the caregiving relationship. These are the notions of giving and facilitation.

In *Dementia Reconsidered*, Kitwood argues that facilitation refers to the carer's awareness and ability to 'enable the person with dementia to do what otherwise he or she would not be able to do by providing those parts of the action—and only those—that are missing' (Kitwood 1997, p. 91). He goes on to suggest that 'a subtle and gentle imagination is called into play. There is a readiness to respond to the gesture which a person with dementia makes … sharing in the creation of meaning and enabling action to occur' (ibid.: 120). Kitwood's notion of facilitation, and particularly his emphasis on the shared creation of meaning, can be extended and considered in a more reciprocal way in terms of how the person with dementia may facilitate others within a care environment. Opportunities for people with dementia to facilitate may be more apparent in a creative setting where, for example, they may initiate a song or offer a movement or gesture which is taken up by others. However, these opportunities for facilitation are also present within caregiving relationships, particularly when dementia care is considered beyond the fulfilment of primary care. An example of people with dementia facilitating others was apparent during one of the initial visits that I made to Mildmay, the care home that I worked with between 2013 and 2015.

During this visit, I sat out in the garden with some of the residents, which was located in a courtyard at the centre of the care home. As we sipped milky tea in the autumn sunlight, I watched a member of care staff push one of the residents around the garden in her wheelchair. As they moved slowly around the edge of the flower beds, the resident advised her on which plants needed tending to and where weeds were growing. As the carer pulled up the weeds, the resident would shake the soil off them and gather them in a neat pile on her lap. During the same visit, I observed one resident teaching another how to crochet in the reception area of the care home. These examples of residents sharing embodied skills and knowledge demonstrated how people with dementia can facilitate the learning of others in a caregiving context. Moreover, they demonstrated the importance of embodied selfhood in understanding the reciprocity of a caregiving relationship, and the capacity of people with dementia to teach others.

In extending Kitwood's notion of facilitation as a technique used by a carer to something that is reciprocal and relational, facilitation may also be seen in the context of the collective, as something that which is attributable to both human and non–human actants. Facilitation within the collective, I suggest, refers to the distributive agency between humans and things which occurs in the moment of their encounter. Latour's description of the behaviour of the collective suggests that 'things' may also act as facilitators in dementia care settings. He suggests that action is always a 'property of associated entities' within a collective, and that in order to understand the action we must at first acknowledge the 'association of actants' that relate to the completion of a goal' (Latour 1999, p. 182). His use of the term *subprogrammes* to explain the particular role of material objects in the completion of the goal, points to the potential of things within relational care in supporting or enabling people with dementia to achieve certain goals. An encounter with a domestic object, for example, may facilitate an embodied action associated with the completion of a particular task, such as dusting or doing the washing up. Encounters with the atmospheric properties of a particular space, such as sounds and smells, may stimulate a different type of embodied activity, such as cooking. Considered in these terms, facilitation points to the agency of non-human artefacts in supporting people with dementia to do things.

Giving, in *Dementia Reconsidered*, alludes to the reciprocity of the caring relationship, by focusing on the ability of people with dementia to demonstrate 'a sensitivity to the moods and feelings of care givers', and of the opportunities to 'express concern, affection or gratitude; make an offer of help, or present a gift' (Kitwood 1997, p. 92). This recognition that people with dementia have much to give is crucial to developing a more relational understanding of dementia care. Kitwood's consideration of mood, feelings and warmth not only indicates the sensing and feeling characteristics of the caregiving relationship, it also suggests that a sensitivity or attunement to the moods and feelings of others may be expressed or received as a gift. The creative context of an arts workshop can increase our awareness of the broader range of gifts on offer from people with dementia, and the act of coming together as a group can support their capacity to give.

The relational context of giving within dementia care also draws attention to the multiple roles that are inhabited by people with dementia and helps to conceive of selfhood as an evolving process. Baldwin and Capstick argue that caregiving relationships are always 'contextually bound' and suggest that a more progressive model of dementia care may consider personhood 'not as a fixed status, but rather as a process grounded in social interaction' (Baldwin and Capstick 2007, p. 182). Rather than being cast solely in the binary roles of 'carer' and 'person with dementia', they argue that personhood should allow people to change and inhabit more than one role at the same time. Their observation is significant because it highlights the inherently relational nature of selfhood, and the wider and composite range of roles that make up the identities of each individual. In addition to being a resident of a care community, a person with dementia may also be a parent or grandparent, a brother or sister, a knowledgeable gardener and a lover of jazz music. By considering identity in terms of a multiple collection of roles, artists may become more aware of the broader range of 'gifts' on offer by people with dementia, and of their ability to make meaningful contributions to a caregiving relationship.

Environmental Aspects of Care

The final component of this relational approach to dementia care is concerned with the way in which the atmospheric and material qualities of the caregiving environment act as relational components of care. In her definition of relational dementia care, Kontos usefully emphasises the 'the centrality of capacities, senses and experiences of bodies to the exercise of human agency and interconnectedness' (Kontos et al. 2017, p. 182). She does not however, consider the role of the material environment. Although I argue later in this chapter that there is a distributive agency between humans and non-humans in a dementia care context, it is first necessary to recognise the inherent liveliness of things within the collective, and to cultivate a sensitivity to their affective potential. In addition to identifying some of the ways in which these environmental features may demonstrate a material and cumulative agency within the collective, my approach is also concerned with cultivating a material awareness of atmosphere, and how components such as lights, sounds and smells and temperatures create an 'affective climate' in the collective.

In his theory of the senses as perceptual systems, the psychologist James Gibson considers the relationship between the embodied self and the environment in terms of 'the way in which the senses obtain information about objects in the world without the intervention of an intellectual process' (Gibson 1966, p. 2). Considering the specific affordances of the animate environment, he explains that: 'The environment consists of opportunities for perception, of available information, of potential stimuli. Not all opportunities are grasped ... but what the environment affords an individual in the way of discrimination is enormous (ibid.: 23)'.

Though drawing his example from the animal world, Gibson's recognition of the affordances of the animate environment and his search for an ecology, rather than a psychology of perception, helps us to consider the dementia care environment in terms of a set of affordances for the embodied self, and an animate ecology of 'things'. Building on Gibson's theory, the human geographer Paul Rodaway suggests that 'the structure and texture of the environment itself ... is a necessary determinant of what is perceived' (Rodaway 2011, p. 20). Rodaway's attention to the structure or ordering of these environmental features, and their determining role in the meaningful construction of place is significant in conceptualising the behaviour of non-human artefacts and how they contribute to the 'feel' of a care environment. This is particularly applicable to the environmental architecture of a care home and how things 'behave' in the construction of public, institutional or homely spaces. For example, the texture, thickness and colour of a carpet underfoot may instantly induce a feeling of homeliness or an association with an institution. The presence of a book case full of books as part of a living room arrangement or access to outdoor garden space may have a homely affect, whereas a fire exit sign or a health and safety poster within a domestic space will create associations with public buildings and work settings. It is the cumulative or collective presence of these non-human artefacts, I argue, that constitute the feel of a care environment and are fundamental to the way it is perceived by the embodied self. The choice and positioning of material objects therefore, has the potential to transform the way in which dementia care is experienced beyond relationships between human beings.

The sociologist Jenny Hockey and colleagues' work on the agency of personal objects in later life is useful in considering the relational qualities of personal possessions, and the emotional animate-ness of things within a care collective. Focusing on the materiality and 'social life of things' within a sheltered housing environment they argue that objects and spaces not only have their own agency but are 'constitutive of the social time and space of later life' (Hockey et al. 2005, p. 139). Their emphasis on the lively persistence of social relations within personal objects encourages us to think about them beyond their sentimental function, as manifestations of caring relationships. Furthermore, their observations on the inherent socialness of personal objects suggests that it is the agential and emotional status of personal things, and their behaviour as lively objects that reveal their relational role in dementia care. By exploring the creative behaviour of things within a theatrical context, and the quality of the interaction between human and the non-human world, I hope to demonstrate some ways in which the creative and affective potential of everyday objects in a care home may be harnessed.

In considering the ways in which the material properties of the space 'behave' within a care collective, it is also important to acknowledge the atmospheric 'climate' of the space. This involves understanding how things that cannot be seen or held, but are sensed, may still have a material presence in the care home. The German philosopher Gernot Böhme suggests that there is an inherent connection between atmosphere and perception and goes as far as defining atmosphere as 'a theory of perception in the full sense of the term, in which perception is understood as the experience of the presence of persons, objects and environments' (Böhme 1993, p. 116). He suggests that atmosphere may only truly be conceptualised however, if 'we succeed in accounting for the peculiar intermediary status of atmospheres between subject and object (ibid.: 114), suggesting that atmosphere may only be become tangible when attributed to a collective of humans and material objects. Similarly, cultural geographer Derek P. McCormack alludes to the 'in-between-ness' of atmosphere as 'something distributed but palpable … a quality of environmental immersion that registers in and through sensing bodies, while also remaining diffuse, in the air, ethereal' (McCormack 2008, p. 414). Following Tim Ingold's conception of atmosphere as both a material and meteorological phenomena (2005), McCormack suggests that an 'affective atmosphere' is best understood as a 'moving materiality' that 'registers differentially the perceptual affordances of sensing bodies' (ibid.).

The notion of atmosphere as a moving materiality not only shows how the atmospheric properties of dementia care environments may be determinants in the way that they are perceived. It also suggests that the atmosphere of a particular care space may shift, alter, or be generated by the collective. McCormack's suggestion that the affective materiality of atmosphere is best registered through the perceptual (or embodied) know-how of humans is useful in conceptualising the relational behaviour of atmosphere within a care environment. It suggests that sounds, smells and other climatic features are brought into being through their contact with humans, and may invite people with dementia to engage with the space in a different way. This has implications for artists who are working in care homes as the sensory affordances of a care home may be more perceptible during an arts workshop. In thinking through how participatory performance might best support relational dementia care, there is an opportunity to explore the atmospheric properties of the space and introduce exercises which support embodied interactions between people and things.

Participatory Performance and Relational Dementia Care

A key consideration of this book is how creative context of an arts workshop can support people with dementia, to, as Jane Bennett puts it, 'do things' in collaboration with the non-human actants in a care environment. If we return to Karen Jürs-Munby's notion of an 'aesthetics of access' in disability-led performance, it is possible to conceive of how the sensory features of a care environment may also become scaffolds which support creative participation. This requires a closer examination of the processes involved in sensory exchange.

In 1992 the biologist David Dusenbury developed the term 'sensory ecology' to articulate his idea that organisms possess a sensory system which is unique to their individual ecology. Sensory ecology refers to the way in which information about the environment is obtained by organisms in a process of sensory exchange. Rather than examining the senses in relation to physiological systems, Dusenbury's theory is concerned with the information that is available from the immediate environment and how this is used by organisms in the process of perception. The idea of information being obtained through a process of sensory exchange can be related to Gibson's argument for the senses as perceptual systems which have 'make us feel and make us perceive', and which have the capacity to obtain information 'without the intervention of an intellectual process' (Gibson 1966, p. 2). In a performance workshop, this information can be received by the body in different ways. A movement exercise may stimulate an exchange of information via the sensation of the foot on the floor, whereas an exercise involving objects could initiate a different type of sensory encounter between the object and the fingertips. An arts project which uses sound or music may encourage residents to engage with the aural properties of a care space, either through the ear or by feeling the vibrations of the sound in another part of the body. The concept of sensory ecology helps artists to think about the creative affordances of a care home, and specifically, what information the care environment offers to residents when they are participating in an arts workshop.

The performance scholar Martin Welton offers an insight into how the sensory properties of a care home may be understood as sensory affordances. In his book *Feeling Theatre,* he takes up James Gibson's distinction between feeling and perception, and considers what the sensory properties of a theatre or rehearsal space might offer a performer as they prepare for a performance. He describes how a performer obtains information from their environment as they move around it. He explains this process as 'the pick up *in* movement of the feeling *about* movement (Welton 2012, p. 3) and 'the socially shaped ways and means of making sense of our surroundings which we take with us from place to place' (ibid.: 106). This process, he argues, is not attributable to a cognitive or emotional type of engagement, but is experienced on an embodied level through movement—what he describes as the 'condition of feeling' (ibid.: 108). Welton's application of Gibson's theory to the rehearsal room is instructive when considering what types of sensory information are available from care environments and it may be 'picked up' by people with dementia on an embodied level. His suggestion that perception is achieved through movement also raises questions about how this information is received through the body as it moves around the space. What type of information is picked up by the body? Do different types of movement lead to different types of exchanges between the body and the space? And how might the notion of a 'feeling engagement' support the body as manifestation of selfhood in dementia care?

The cultural anthropologist Thomas Csordas preceded Pia Kontos' suggestion that 'the body is a significant dimension of selfhood' in dementia by arguing that it should be understood as 'a condition where culture and self are grounded' (Csordas 1993, p. 136). Drawing on Maurice Merleau-Ponty's work on the body as field of perception, Csordas theorised a 'paradigm of embodiment' in which perception was considered less as a cognitive process and more as a type of bodily engagement. Csordas' insistence that embodied experience is the starting point for analysing human participation in the world and his question: 'how we can pay attention with and to our bodies?', foregrounds the role of the body in making sense of a care space, and the information that is received by the body through movement. It leads me to question how different types of movement in an arts workshop might induce 'feeling engagements' with a care space, and how this condition of feeling may be experienced by people with limited mobility, who are unable to travel around the care home on foot.

Considering feeling as both an emotional state and a physical sensation, Welton suggests that the two are not easily separable as they are 'both specified in relation to our physical and social environments' (Welton 2012, p. 9). Instead, he suggests that a perceptual or sensing ecology exists 'on a continuum with an affective one' to the extent that 'the two are not entirely distinguishable' (ibid.). This notion of a sensory-affective continuum suggests that a person with dementia's bodily experiences may exist on a continuum with their emotional ones, and that the distribution of physical sensation and emotional affect may shift with changes in the care environment. This idea is central to the creative approach outlined in this book, which is concerned with how creative practice can invoke different types of 'feeling engagements' with a care space. I am interested in how the sensory affordances of the care home may be identified, and whether these environmental features are experienced differently in an arts workshop to how they would be in an everyday context. In other words, how is the process of 'getting a feel for something' affected by the creative context of the workshop? And how might creative practice draw attention to the sensory affordances of a seemingly ordinary environmental feature?

A sensory ecology for creative practice can draw attention to the broader range of creative possibilities available from and within a care space, and the capacity of material objects as a source of information or action. Gibson's description of the properties of the animate environment is particularly instructive here. He argues that all objects within a living ecology possess their own energy and status as a 'reflecting body' which has the capacity to 'radiate structure or information' (Gibson 1966, p. 15). Using the term 'contact mechanisms' to describe the consequences of human contact with these objects, he alludes to Latour's argument that material objects 'are not a neutral carrier of human will' and that 'each artefact has its script, its potential to take hold of a passer-by and force them to play roles in its story' (Latour 1999, p. 177).

Gibson's argument that objects radiate information not only prompts artists to consider the lively status of personal or everyday objects in a performance workshop. It also suggests that these objects might offer something particular in the moment of their encounter with humans. An example of this might be when an object from the care home is improvised as a prop or an item of clothing belonging to a resident is used as a piece of costume. Furthermore, when considered in terms of feeling theatre, the notion of contact mechanisms may be understood more broadly as an encounter between the body and the space, which occurs during movement. Welton explains this process using the example of an actor's foot moving across the boards of the stage:

> The actor senses herself in contact with the boards of the stage through the sole of her foot, and feels the affordance for her performance offered by the composite set of relations she establishes in moving across them. The boards themselves might be bare, but in sensing the affordance that they offer her, she experiences once more a sense of her nestedness, and is returned to something of the experience of the original environment of the rehearsal room. (Welton 2012, p. 124)

Welton's description of the relationship between feeling and movement in the rehearsal room illustrates how the material affordances of a care home may be experienced by people with dementia during movement. It suggests that the sensations that are induced during movement may help to create sense of place, whether it be a place from reality, memory or from imagination. The feeling of 'nestedness' that is achieved by the actor through the sensation of their foot on the floor is pertinent to me as a practitioner, in terms of how the sensory properties of floors, objects or surfaces in the care space may offer something meaningful to participants. It also encourages artists who are working in care homes to consider how the creative context of a workshop can invite tactile encounters with everyday spaces. 'Wandering behaviour' is commonly understood to be a symptom of dementia, particularly for those who have moved to care homes and are getting used to new surroundings. However, an increased focus on the experience of dementia has led researchers, particularly dance therapists, to question the nature and definition of 'wandering' as something aimless or directionless, and to consider it instead as a purposeful journey between two places. Mary Marshall and Kate Allan develop this idea in their book *Dementia: Walking not Wandering* (2006), where they challenge medical perspectives on wandering and celebrate walking as a way of creating a sense of place in dementia care. Welton's notion of movement as a process of perception supports the idea of walking as a purposeful act and a way of creating a sense of place. He explains that 'walking shares with making and working that crucial element of the body and the mind with the world, of knowing the world through the body and the body through the world' (Welton 2012, p. 120).

The idea of walking as a means of 'knowing the world' raises questions about the possibilities of creative practice in supporting the 'wandering behaviour' of people with dementia. This could occur by creating opportunities for movement which respond to the need that these residents have to travel between different places. For example, an artist might support walking as a purposeful act by walking *with* a resident with dementia, engaging with their patterns of movement and validating their journey between different places. Similarly, the use of music might help to validate repetitious journeys between different places in a care home. By considering walking as a means of knowing the world, artists who work in care settings may develop strategies for supporting the personal habits and embodied practices of people with dementia as creative acts in their own right.

Objects and Improvisation

James Gibson suggests that the environment provides opportunities for perception. A care environment can also provide opportunities for improvisation in a participatory performance context. For artists working in care homes, developing an awareness of the material properties of a care space can increase their understanding of how they are experienced by people with dementia through improvisatory encounters. Following Latour's idea that humans and non-humans co-exist as a network of *actants* (Bennett 2010, viii), Jane Bennett offers a theory of vibrant materialism, which is concerned with cultivating 'sensory attentiveness' (ibid.: 15) to non-human forces operating outside and inside the human body. An awareness of the vitality of matter, she suggests, is essential in helping us to understand the potency of the material environment, and the 'fuller range of the nonhuman power circulating around and within human bodies' (ibid.: ix).

Bennett's attention to the materiality of things is fundamental to a sensory approach in considering how props, personal objects and other non-human artefacts may increase the accessibility of an arts workshop for people with dementia. As a theatre practitioner, it encourages me to consider the way in which the material components of care spaces are experienced sensorially through the embodied self, and what they offer a participant by way of information or exchange. By raising the status of things, and distributing agency between human and non-human bodies, Bennett argues, vibrant materialism could 'raise a safety net … for those humans [who] do not conform to a particular model of personhood' (ibid.: 13). I intend to test her suggestion by exploring the vibrant status of material objects in performance workshops and how they support embodied forms of participation.

Bennett uses the term 'Thing-Power' to describe the potential of objects as vibrant things which command attention in their own right. Things, as opposed to objects, she argues, possess an 'energetic vitality' (ibid.: 2). They have the potential to make things happen and a 'tendency to persist in excess of their associations with human beings' (ibid.). Her notion of Thing-Power suggests that the non-human artefacts of a care environment may have a type of agency which supports the creative participation of people with dementia. The idea that objects can become vibrant things, which are energetically connected to human bodies, is helpful in understanding the creative potential of human and non-human collaborations in an arts workshop. It also raises questions as to how and when everyday objects in a care home acquire the status of things. Are 'things', for example, objects that belong to the residents, or do they extend to domestic objects, furniture, props or even objects from memory and the imagination? If 'thing power' does exist, how might arts practitioners harness it and use it in a creative way? And what might the creative context of a workshop offer in revealing or unlocking their agency?

In cultivating an awareness of the vitality of things, I have become aware of the theatricality of the moment in which an object takes on a 'thing-like' status and is experienced by a participant as remarkable. Bennett describes this as 'the moment when the object becomes the Other and the subject experiences the object as uncanny' (ibid.). For Sarah Hopfinger, thing-power is a resource that can be embedded within a devising process and used to explore 'our ecological connectedness with the nonhuman' (Hopfinger 2018, p. 499). Reflecting on *Wild Life,* the intergenerational performance project where performers 'worked with and as vibrant matter', she describes how they engaged in 'playful activities … with non-human materials' (ibid.: 501). These activities included 'working with stones, rocks, matches, fire, smoke, buckets and water' (ibid.) and exploring 'how movement arises from being in contact with specific textures, colours, smells or temperatures (ibid.). She describes a rehearsal when performers flung or slid stones across the stage floor, standing at different spots around the circular performance space. The company gradually become more adept at intuiting how far the stones would travel and where they would land in the space:

> The human performers were fully committed to, and wholly focused on, the task of sliding stones, which meant that their ideas about how to slide the stones were able to emerge immanently from the movements of the stones: the movements of the different humans were entangled with the movements and tendencies of the different stones as well as how the other humans slid their stones. (Ibid.: 512)

What Hopfinger seems to be getting at here is the way in which the quality of the performers' throwing movements (speed, direction, force, gesture, posture) was led by the objects themselves rather than human instruction. Examples of objects acquiring 'thing-power' can also be apparent when the theatrical context of the workshop requires objects to take on a role in a story. This potential was apparent during an improvisation project that I led with performers who had early stage dementia and their partners. There were occasions in our workshops where personal objects that belonged to the participants became 'lively' during creative exercises. There were instances, for example, where a watch, a pocket diary and a hair comb became props that were used by a fictional character in a scene. At other times, objects were improvised as things that were different to their intended purpose. In another exercise, the participants passed a scarf around the circle and imagined that it was something else by miming an action that was associated with the new object.

An awareness of Thing-Power increases an artist's understanding of the creative potential of objects in a dementia care setting, and how this can emerge through collaborations between humans and non-humans. In turn, these sorts of exercises can increase their awareness of the creative strategies that people with dementia use to participate in arts workshops. These strategies, which do not rely on long-term memory, include improvisation, imagination and embodied interactions with things. In considering the effect of Thing-Power, Bennett proposes that the materiality of things is 'as much about force and energy as entity and matter' (Bennett, 201, p. 20). This suggests that it is not just the co-existence of humans and non-humans, but what happens when they come together that is significant in understanding how a dementia care collective works in practice. The force or energy that occurs during the encounter between humans and things will be considered throughout this book in terms of how the non-human components of care environments support people with dementia to do things.

When rejecting the humanist distinctions of subject and object, and the notion of humanity as 'the sole or ultimate wellspring of agency' (ibid.: 30), Bennett uses Deleuze and Guattari's concept of the assemblage in order to consider the combined potential of humans and things. She suggests that agency is something that occurs as a result of an encounter between human and non-human matter. An assemblage, in Bennett's terms, is made up of an 'ad hoc grouping of diverse elements' (ibid.: 23), which have a 'distributive agency' and whose coming together increases their capacity for action. Her notion of distributive agency is particularly significant to my approach, in terms of the relational exchanges that take place between people and things in an arts workshop. In the same way that Goodley and Runswick-Cole outline how a 'dis/human' collective functions as an interdependent community of human and non-human assemblages, Bennett's concept of distributive agency points to the way that agency may be distributed between a participant and a material object in a continual process of exchange. Distributive agency removes the pressure for people with dementia to negotiate a care environment autonomously and shows how non-human actants can increase their capacity.

Addressing the agentic balance of the human-object assemblage, and what she considers to be a human tendency to 'understate the degree to which people, animals, artefacts, technologies and elemental forces share powers and operate in dissonant conjunction with each other' (ibid.: 35), Bennett suggests that greater weight should be given to actions that originate from things. She uses the Chinese notion of *shi* to describe this type of action that originates 'not in human initiative but instead results from the very disposition of things' (ibid.). The notion of *shi* speaks to the improvisatory potential of things, and to objects that stimulate spontaneous sensory encounters. A theatre workshop can draw attention to the improvisatory potential of these objects, supporting their transformation into 'things' which offer something particular in the moment of their encounter with humans. Moreover, the notion of *shi* helps artists to understand how everyday objects, when employed in a theatrical way, may support people with dementia to participate in different ways. For example, workshops which involve sensory interactions with certain props may evoke embodied memories and actions that are connected to the home. The sensation of water in a washing up bowl, or the feel of a feather duster, could evoke embodied memories and actions that are associated with domestic tasks. Alternatively, the weight and texture of work tools may feel familiar to someone who is accustomed to manual labour. A sensory approach enables practitioners to consider improvisation beyond an exchange that takes place between humans and to consider the role of non-humans in supporting the creative participation of people with dementia. It draws attention to the affective potential of things, and how the feelings that are induced through their interaction with humans can lead to different forms of participation.

Bringing the Weather Indoors

The final part of this chapter explores sensory ecology in relation to the atmospheric affordances of the workshop space. Using Welton's image of 'bringing the weather indoors', it considers the climate of the workshop space as something that is both sensed and generated collectively by the participants. I suggest that a sensory approach to practice, which draws on the climatic properties of the space, may broaden artists' awareness of the material status of atmosphere within a care collective.

Welton proposes that 'getting a feel for how it goes' involves a process of attuning to atmospheric shifts as much as material ones (Welton 2012, p. 126). Considering the overlap of climate with felt experience, he describes the significance of weather as something that is both ever-present and 'an experience which can be shared between humans' (ibid.). This shared sense of place, he suggests, which is cultivated through 'feeling or imagining atmospheric conditions' (ibid.) is particularly significant to theatrical feeling.

Welton's reflections on atmosphere draw attention to how it has been somewhat neglected within participatory theatre research. It prompts me to consider how a sensory approach may reveal the atmospheric conditions of the space itself, and how different climates may be cultivated collectively between participants and things. In considering the nature of atmosphere as something that is both meteorological and generative, McCormack proposes that it is both 'processual, distributed, and sensed', suggesting that atmosphere is both material enough to be registered and distributed through humans, while existing simultaneously as something that is 'diffuse, in the air, ethereal' (McCormack 2008, p. 414). This conception of atmosphere as material, yet ethereal, is significant to this ecological approach to practice, in terms of how artists go about cultivating an atmospheric mindfulness in workshops. This involves understanding how atmospheres not only inhabit a particular space, but are also generated and distributed by participants. Welton's association of theatrical feeling with the act of feeling or imagining atmospheric conditions also raises an interesting consideration for practice, not only as to how a sensory approach may cultivate different atmospheres, but also how an arts workshop may tap into the atmospheric conditions of particular spaces.

In some instances, these subtle manifestations of atmosphere are more tangible at the beginning of the session, before the main activity has started. In 2012 I took part in a sound and movement project that was designed for people with dementia and run by artists from the Trinity Laban Conservatoire in London. During a vocal warm up exercise which took place at the start of the session, the artist-facilitator Natasha Lohan invited participants to focus on the rhythm of their breath and on the sounds that were audible within and beyond the room. As we listened to the distant rumble of the traffic, the sound of the central heating system and the faint hum of conversation in the next room, the room became very still. The act of listening closely together had created a shared engagement with the atmospheric properties of the workshop space. Similarly, I observed how the collective layering of sounds that were generated during the vocal warm up echoed and reverberated around the space, distributing a particular atmosphere which changed the feeling of the space and lingered long after the exercise had finished. This exercise was repeated at the beginning of every session, partly to warm up our voices, but also to engage with the space we were working in and to bring our attention to the way that it could be encountered through sound and movement.

Alluding to the materiality of atmospheric sound, Gibson remarks that the 'correspondence of sound waves to their source means that the information about an event is physically present in the air around the event' (Gibson 1966, p. 13). His ecological interpretation of sound helps me to consider how the sounds emitted from the ambient environment, and from the participants' voices, generated an atmosphere that was both familiar, and materially present as well as existing as something that was 'in the air' and unique to that particular moment in the workshop.

Böhme's argument for atmosphere as a theory of perception is also instructive in understanding its role in participatory arts practice. In his attempt to 'liberate' atmosphere from a 'subjective-objective dichotomy' and the notion that atmosphere is registered solely through the body (Böhme 1993, p. 121), he echoes Gibson's thoughts on the emitting disposition of objects, suggesting that atmosphere is registered and radiated through the quality of things. Atmospheres, he suggests, are not just created by things, but are in themselves 'thing like' in that their presence is articulated though their atmospheric properties. It is 'the form of a thing', Böhme suggests, that imbues atmosphere with its affective status or capacity and 'exerts an external effect' (ibid.). His proposal that atmosphere is not only inhabited but exerted through things suggests that the atmosphere of a care space may be perceived through everyday things, as well as being conceived or produced collectively and creatively in an arts workshop. Additionally, Böhme's insistence that atmosphere is something 'that proceeds from, or is created by 'constellations' of things and persons' (122) helps us to understand atmosphere as a creation of the collective. The shared cultivation of atmosphere in a participatory arts context may also play a vital role in the way that it is perceived.

This chapter outlined a relational approach to dementia care which was inspired by posthumanism. It considered what the care environment can offer people with dementia, and how 'non-human' elements such as objects, spaces and atmospheres might act as 'agents' in a caregiving relationship. Considering how people with dementia interact with the care environment at an embodied level, it proposed that care home residents might act in confederation with the non-human actants of a care environment, and that creative practice might increase their opportunities to do so. The second half of this book puts this idea into practice, exploring the relationship between performance and the care environment.

In the following chapter, I consider some of the ways in which care environments are constructed through sound. Offering an audio analysis of a care home dining room, I explore sound as a creative affordance which can help residents to establish a sense of place, as well as connecting them to other significant times and places outside the care home. The chapter also interrogates practices of listening and how the 'sonorous bodies' of participants, in a performance context, can change the way that a care space is perceived.

Note

1. Kitwood outlined six psychological requirements that needed to be met in order for people with dementia to achieve a high standard of person-centred care (see 1997, 82).

References

Baldwin, C., & Capstick, A. (Eds.). (2007). *Tom Kitwood on Dementia: A Reader and Critical Commentary*. New York: Open University Press.

Bartlett, R., & O'Connor, D. (2010). *Broadening the Dementia Debate: Towards Social Citizenship*. Bristol: Policy Press.

Beach, M., & Inui, T. (2006). Relationship-Centred Care: A Constructive Reframing. *Journal of General Internal Medicine, 21*, 3–8.

Bennett, J. (2010). *Vibrant Matter: A Political Ecology of Things*. Durham: Duke University Press.

Böhme, G. (1993). Atmosphere as the Fundamental Concept of a New Aesthetics. *Thesis Eleven, 36*, 113–126.

Csordas, T. (1993). Somatic Modes of Attention. *Cultural Anthropology, 8*(2), 135–156.

Gibson, J. (1966). *The Senses Considered as Perceptual Systems*. London: George Allan and Unwin Press.

Goodley, D. (2014). *Dis/ability Studies: Theorising Disablism and Ableism*. London: Routledge.

Hockey, J., Penhale, B., & Sibley, D. (2005). Environments of Memory: Home, Space, Later Life and Grief. In J. Davidson, L. Bondi, & M. Smith (Eds.), *Emotional Geographies* (pp. 135–146). Aldershot: Ashgate Press.

Hopfinger, S. (2018). Intergenerational Performance Ecology: A Practice-Based Approach. *Research in Drama Education, 23*(4), 499–516.

Ingold, T. (2005). The eye of the storm: visual perception and the weather. *Visual Studies, 20*, 98–104.

Kitwood, T. (1997). *Dementia Reconsidered*. Milton Keynes: Open University Press.

Kontos, P. (2004). Ethnographic Reflections on Selfhood, Embodiment and Alzheimer's Disease. *Aging and Society, 24*(6), 829–849.

Kontos, P. (2005). Embodied Selfhood in Alzheimer's Disease: Rethinking Person-Centred Care. *Dementia, 4*(4), 553–570.

Kontos, P., Miller, K., & Kontos, A. (2017). Relational Citizenship: Supporting Embodied Selfhood and Relationality in Dementia Care. *Sociology of Health and Illness, 39*(2), 182–198.

Latour, B. (1999). *Pandora's Hope: Essays on the Reality of Science Studies*. Cambridge, MA: Harvard University Press.

Marshall, M., & Allan, K. (Eds.). (2006). *Dementia: Walking Not Wandering – Fresh Approaches to Understanding and Practice*. London: Hawker.

McCormack, D. (2008). Engineering Affective Atmospheres on the Moving Geographies of the 1897 Andree Expedition. *Cultural Geographies, 15*, 413–431.

Nolan, M. (2006). *The Senses Framework: Improving Care for Older People Through a Relationship-Centred Approach*. Getting Research into Practice (GRiP) Report No 2. Project Report, University of Sheffield.

Nolan, M., Davies, S., Brown, J., Keady, J., & Nolan, J. (2004). Beyond Person-Centred Care: A New Vision for Gerontological Nursing. *International Journal of Older People Nursing, 13*(3a), 45–53.

Rodaway, P. (2011). *Sensuous Geographies.* London: Routledge.

Welton, M. (2012). *Feeling Theatre.* London: Palgrave Macmillan.

PART II

Performance and the Care Environment

CHAPTER 5

'A Poetics of Sound': Towards an Aural Re-imagining of a Care Home Dining Room

> When insomnia … is increased through irritation caused by city noises … I can recover my calm by living the metaphors of the ocean … I dream an abstract-concrete daydream. My bed is a small boat lost at sea; that sudden whistling is the wind in the sails. On every side the air is filled with the sound of furious klaxoning. I talk to myself to give myself cheer: there there, your skiff is holding its own, you are safe in your stone boat. Sleep in spite of the storm. Sleep in the storm. Sleep in your own courage, happy to be a man who is assailed by wind and the wave. And I fall asleep, lulled by the noise of Paris. (Bachelard 1992, p. 28)

In imagining the noise of Paris at night time as the sound of the sea, the philosopher Gaston Bachelard invites us to hear by imagination, attending to what is there and what is not. This 'space of imagination', which enables him to fuse the 'concrete' noise of the city with the 'abstract' sounds of the sea is what he calls 'inhabited space' and forms the basis of his 1964 work *The Poetics of Space*. His oft-quoted declaration that 'inhabited space transcends geometric space' (Ibid., p. 47) summarises his proposal that space is constructed as much from daydreams and memories, as the 'geometric lines and borders' that make up buildings and cities. *The Poetics of Space* is built around the sentimental image of a childhood home. This home is a symbol of security from the outside world, a haven for secrets which are locked in wardrobes and drawers, and a place which escapes the cramped conditions of the city by rising up to the sky and down into the earth.

N. Hatton, *Performance and Dementia*,
https://doi.org/10.1007/978-3-030-51077-0_5

The contradictions between Bachelard's house of the imagination and a care home are numerous. To start with, the verticality of his three-story house which has steps stretching down into the cellar and up to the attic are unlikely to feature in a care home, or be accessible to residents, who are often confined to one floor. The old drawers and wardrobes that Bachelard associates with intimacy and charm are homely objects that are rarely to be found in care home bedrooms. Furthermore, his romanticisation of locks and keys as gateways to places where humans can keep or hide their secrets take on a very different meaning when they are associated with safety management and, in some cases, preventing residents from getting out. However, Bachelard's re-imagining of everyday space and his attention to the intimate and intricate composition of domestic spaces provides a valuable foundation on which to explore the everyday creativity of a care home. In particular, his re-imagining of city noises as the sounds of the sea is significant to my interest in sound and the creative potential of care spaces. It poses a question about whether the everyday sounds of a care home may be understood in terms of their affordances. Care spaces are heavily constituted by sound, and the juxtaposition of different sounds in communal spaces can be a powerful institutional signifier. Additionally, sound can be a disruptive influence when running an arts project in a care homes as it can dominate the space. My interest in the relational possibilities of sound has prompted me to consider how the sounds of a care home may be 're-imagined' or perceived differently through creative practice.

This chapter is an aural exploration of a care home dining room. Exploring the interplay between environmental, ambient and musical sounds, it poses two questions: What can sound teach us about space in a care home? Can sound support the possibilities of a care home as a creative space? The focus of the chapter is a sound project and installation that I created with residents at 20–26 Mildmay Park over a 6-week period. 20–26 Mildmay Park (referred to as 'Mildmay' hereafter) is a care service in North London which is run by Notting Hill Genesis (previously known as Notting Hill Housing). It operates as part of three interconnected sites that offer different levels of supported living. This includes supporting older adults (65+), some who are living with dementia and some younger adults with physical and learning difficulties. It is a domiciliary care facility—which means that the residents receive some form of personal care but are supported to live as independently as possible. The residents from Mildmay come from a diverse range of age groups, social and cultural backgrounds, as well as having a broad range of access needs. This range was reflected in the make-up of the group that took part in the project. There were 14 participants that took part over the six weeks with a core group of seven residents that attended each week. These residents ranged in age between 55 and 86 and there was a mixture of cognitively able adults, people living with mild to moderate dementia, and some younger adults with learning difficulties. As a result of this, the preference for what we did during the project was quite diverse. The range in ages, interests and abilities of the participants prompted an important line of inquiry about personal taste, and how this informs creative practice in care homes. This is considered in detail in the following chapter.

The project involved weekly, two-hour workshops in the dining room which were facilitated by me, the sound designer Jamie Flockton, and three applied theatre students from the Royal Central School of Speech and Drama—Jessie Sherman, Stella Nouli and Sara Athans. It culminated in the presentation of the sound installation and an informal performance of poetry, singing and short scenes to an audience of residents and care staff. This was followed by a celebration with music, tea and cakes.

The creative team met before the first session in order to discuss the aims of the project. We all agreed that a primary aim was to provide an opportunity for the residents to socialise and express themselves creatively. I had discovered from volunteering at the care home that many of the residents had participated in music and theatre throughout their lives (some of them professionally), and some expressed a desire for singing and readings plays. We felt that it was important to provide opportunities for this, as well as exploring the creative possibilities of sound together. Consequently, sessions were structured to include song and script work based on music and plays that the residents told us about. Usually, the plan for the following week's session would be shaped around things that we had found out about the residents in the previous week.

Exploring Everyday Sound

In planning a series of sound-based exercises for the project, I was interested in finding opportunities to explore the creative possibilities of the space. Working with Jamie Flockton was an integral part of this process as this was a departure from my usual way of working with sound. Although I use sound in a lot of my participatory performance work, I had never worked directly with the sounds of the rehearsal space before. Nor had I led projects where sound was the artistic focus of the project. Similarly, though Jamie and I had worked together before, our work had always followed a more conventional process of him composing and sourcing sounds for a performance. Rather than designing a piece to support the final performance, the idea was that he would bring along different sounds each week which we would use as a stimulus for the workshops. For example, one session had a sea theme, which we introduced by playing sea shanties and a soundscape of the ocean. Having Jamie participate in each session also enabled us to record the voices of the residents and the sounds of the room in a cumulative fashion, with a view to creating an installation for the space. In addition to a creating a piece of performance that was inspired by a range of different audio locations, we felt that a group sound piece was something that had the potential to endure in between the sessions and after the project had finished. For example, it could be played during mealtimes and activities, by residents in their bedrooms, or to visitors and family members. I hoped it would also be a way of engaging the participants with dementia, who could contribute in a range of ways without the pressure of remembering what we did week to week. Recording every session enabled us to capture their words, songs and sounds in a literal way and encouraged us to create a sound piece which was not bound by the conventions of a linear story.

In considering the aesthetic value of sound-based practice with people with dementia, I was inspired by the work of the Canadian artist Aynsley Moorhouse who made audio recordings with her father in the weeks leading up to his death. In *Turning* (2012), Moorhouse uses her father's repeated words, the sounds of the care facility and their conversations to create what she describes as 'an intimate engagement with my father's experience with dementia' (Moorhouse 2014). The effect is a soundscape of fragments, singing and sounds which seem to reflect the embodied experience of her father's dementia, but also capture the creativity of his fragmented memories and observations. By capturing the participants' voices in an ongoing fashion, I hoped that we could create something which was faithful to their contributions, as well as drawing attention to their artistic value. Additionally, many residents seemed to be interested in the process of making individual audio recordings. One woman, Pauline, would hold her hand out in front of her when Jamie went around the circle with the microphone as if to suggest that she was keen to go next. Some group members expressed pleasure in hearing their voices on the recording and smiled with recognition as they were played back to them.

The experience made me realise that the process of making the recordings and listening to them together in the workshops each week was as much of a creative act as the final sound piece that we created at the end of the project.

In the same way that the residents who took part had diverse preferences for the types of activities that we did, I anticipated that they would interpret and respond to sound in different ways. In a Japanese study which explored how men and women with dementia respond to environmental sounds differently, Koji Nagahata and colleagues observed that the 'clashing of pots and pans' was a familiar sound to many of the women who took part in the study. The men, on the other hand, 'did not react' to these sounds or remarked that it 'just represented noise' (2004, p. 2). Aside from matters of taste, and the diverse cultural and gender associations that are attached to domestic sounds, their study suggests that there are also issues of health and comfort attached to using sound in a care home. Environmental noise, high pitched sounds and loud noises in particular, can be distressing or disorienting for people with dementia. Furthermore, there is evidence to suggest that dementia can change the way in which people interpret the sounds around them. For example, the dementia researcher Jan Dewing suggests that Alzheimer's Disease 'generally result(s) in progressive and significant changes in how people interpret what they see, hear, taste, feel and smell' and that 'agitation can be caused from 'sensory overload or under load from noise' (2009, p. 35). Similarly, the environmental gerontologist Rosemary Bakker suggests that though many people with dementia continue to retain normal hearing, they can 'lose the ability to interpret what they hear accurately' (2003, p. 48). I was aware that some participants may find certain environmental sounds uncomfortable and I wanted to make sure that the more 'active' soundscapes didn't cause discomfort or distress. However, I didn't want this caution to limit us to using only relaxing sounds. Although I wanted to create opportunities for relaxation and reflection, I also wanted to bring in sounds which were stimulating and created associations with other places. It was therefore important that we had a varied selection of soundscapes to bring into the workshop, and a flexible approach, so that we could change tack if there was any discomfort with the sounds we were using.

Jamie prepared a range of contrasting soundscapes for the first sessions including natural soundscapes and urban pieces that were associated with travel and cities. By bringing along a selection of sounds that originated from outside the care home, we hoped that we could create connections to other places that residents enjoyed or remembered. For example, a lot of the participants responded enthusiastically to sounds of the sea, which evoked memories of different places and events. For Dora, the sea soundscape reminded her of traveling over to England from Ireland in a boat and feeling seasick. Elena told us about growing up in Malta and watching the fishing boats 'bobbing up and down on the ocean'. Pauline recalled going on seaside holidays in Britain with her parents. The sea soundscape was a good example of how sounds which belonged to outside the care home could be used to evoke other places and times that were significant in the participants' lives. This discovery felt important in understanding the relationality of the care community and how residents' individual experiences of the care home are shaped by other significant places, experiences and events.

What was more challenging was finding out how we might work creatively with the everyday sounds of the dining room. By engaging creatively with these sounds, as opposed to competing with them, I wanted to know whether they could be 'heard' in a different way. I also wanted to explore the possibilities of listening to these sounds as a shared sensory experience. In order to do this, it was first necessary to explore the acoustic properties of the dining room, and how they contributed to a unique soundscape.

The Care Home Soundscape

In his idealised image of the old childhood home Bachelard invites us to imagine the acoustic characteristics of its different rooms. The voices that are heard on the stairs, he suggests, will sound different if they are heard from the bedroom, and the shape, size and properties of each space will create a different aural experience for the listener: 'The old house, for those who know how to listen, is a sort of geometry of echoes. The voices of the past do not sound the same in the big room as in the little bed chamber, and calls on the stairs have yet another sound' (Bachelard 1992, p. 60). My own audio experiences of care homes are not so easily associated with a geometry of echoes. They are more associated with a network of noise in which televisions, door entry systems, loud music, and conversations overlap and compete. Similarly, in her study of one-to-one arts practices in care homes Caoimhe McAvinchey observed that 'the sounds of televisions on different stations, radios, doors closing and the hum of conversation were a constant soundscape' (McAvinchey 2013, p. 366). Indeed, there is evidence to suggest that the continual audio overload in a care home can be one of the most disorienting changes in the transition from a family home to residential care. Bakker observes that 'many people living in care homes and nursing facilities are subjected to loud and disturbing sounds of alarms, call bells, and overhead paging systems throughout their day' and that noise can be 'a known stressor, especially to people with dementia (Bakker 2003, p. 48). This is particularly true of communal areas such as dining rooms and lounge spaces, which often function simultaneously as multipurpose spaces. However, Bachelard's suggestion that the physical and architectural properties of these spaces affect the way in which sound is received is useful in considering the creative potential of these everyday sounds, and how space affects how the sound is received. A key question when planning the project was how we might explore the audio possibilities of the room without causing additional disruption or discomfort to residents.

The workshops ran straight after lunchtime which meant we were usually setting up as residents were finishing their meals. This was an interesting time to work in the space as the acoustic properties of the room were most prominent. As Jamie tested his speakers, the music would get swallowed up by the clatter of cutlery, and the blare of the television. I wanted to become familiar with these noises and the relationship they had to the room, for example, how sound travelled across different surfaces, the level of echo and the presence of background noise from outside the space. In addition to understanding what we were up against, I wanted to explore how we might use these sounds in our project. The hum of the kitchen fan, the noise of traffic outside, voices from the corridors, cutlery, and shoes on the laminate floor, were all sounds that we noted over the six weeks, and though these sounds were distracting at times, the audio practices of lunchtime at Mildmay became a familiar part of our sessions. This is not to say that the sounds of the room were exclusively unpleasant sounds. There were also some sounds which we heard which challenged the association of the room as an institutional space. These included conversations between friends, music, the laughter of care staff, and the sound of the birds singing outside the patio doors. However, I was interested in the less palatable environmental sounds and whether we might be able to experience them as something different.

For this task, I found myself returning to Bachelard's notion of imagined space, which invited me to re-imagine noisy night time Paris as the roar of the sea. Although it is a highly romanticised image, the concept of imagined space offers the possibility of re-imaging unpleasant sounds as something else, through close listening or manipulation. It raises questions about the aesthetic potential of everyday sound, and how the residents might respond creatively to the noises of the room. The clattering of pots and pans in the adjoining kitchen for example, or the noise of plates being washed may evoke positive associations with home and domestic activities. By cultivating an aesthetic understanding of these everyday sounds, I hoped that we could explore the possibilities of the dining room as a creative space. Bachelard's delight in the echoes of an old house stem partly from its architectural characteristics, but also from the quality of its sounds, and the ability to imagine them as something different. In considering the unique soundscape of the dining room at Mildmay, I began to consider how these everyday sounds may be used to create new audio experiences within the room.

In understanding the relationship between the sounds we brought in and the everyday sounds of the room, it useful to consider some spatial and theoretical aspects of sound. In sound theory, particularly in film, the term *diegesis* is used to describe the different types of sound that are heard in film. Film theorist Barbara Flueckiger describes diegesis as 'the space-time continuum in which a fictional action takes place' (Flueckiger 2009, p. 168) and consequently, 'diegetic sounds' are those which take place inside the fictional world of the film, such as dialogue or an actor firing a gun. 'Non-diegetic sounds' are audio elements from outside the fictional world of the film, such as atmospheric music or sound effects. In reality, these distinctions are complicated by a number of variables, including whether the source of the diegetic sound is visible in the frame. There are also occasions when non-diegetic sounds, such as atmospheric music, can enter the 'real space' of the film. This is particularly prevalent in avant-garde films where, for example, an actor may comment on a sound which originated from outside the fictional world of the film. However, these definitions are useful in considering the relationship between the sounds we brought into the workshop and the everyday sounds of the space.

In exploring the potential of everyday sound in a care home, I must also acknowledge some of the challenges and limitations attached to this work. In the same way that Bachelard has been criticised for sentimentalising the childhood home, I am cautious of overstating the possibilities of working creatively with the sounds of a care home. The sounds that we heard were often loud, unpleasant and disruptive, preventing us from hearing each other and swallowing up the external sounds we brought into the space. Over the course of the six weeks these disruptions included a workman coming to fix a ceiling light, a staff meeting which took place on the other side of the room, and (most frequently) the sound of staff clearing up the kitchen at the end of lunch. Additionally, in exploring the creative potential of these everyday sounds I was aware that people would respond to them in different ways. The noise of pots and pans clashing in the kitchen may be a familiar and positive sound to some people (like the Japanese women in Nagahata's study), but it may evoke negative associations in others. This is particularly pertinent to domestic environments and a criticism of *The Poetics of Space* is that the childhood home is not always a positive place to remember.

Natalia Cecire evokes Lefebvre's criticisms of Bachelard, arguing that the sentimental rendering of the old house grants it the status of a natural space which is unearned. This is illustrated through his recurrent image of the nest which Cecire suggests 'becomes an allegory for the home ... the birds and their habitat become a metonym of nature, such that the human home is itself granted the status of nature, absolute space' (2011, p. 2). Cecire's reservations are useful in understanding the limitations of Bachelard's approach in a care home context. In particular, it suggests that sentimentalising domestic sounds may not be appropriate or enjoyable for everyone. However, the process of identifying the care home soundscape offered a starting point for engaging with the everyday sounds of the room and discovering which sounds the group wanted to explore. I would like to discuss two examples from practice in order to illustrate how we attempted to engage with these everyday sounds. The first is a vocal warm-up exercise which was repeated each week, and the second is a session which was dedicated to creating soundscapes from objects in the room.

Sound, Listening and Material Imagination

Over several essays, Bachelard distinguishes between two different types of imagination: the material and the formal. In an essay entitled 'Earth and Reveries of Will' he explains that the formal imagination is connected to visually perceived images, which are associated with memory and psychological imagination. He explains, it is 'the perception of images which determines the process of the imagination ... we begin by seeing things, then we imagine them; we combine through the imagination, fragments of perceived reality, memories of experienced reality....' (Bachelard 2002, p. 12). Material imagination, on the other hand, is associated with images of matter, and is concretised through a conscious engagement with the material world: '...in addition to the images of form there are ... images of matter. Vision names them but the hand knows them' (Ibid., p. 11). Bachelard's ideas are expanded further by the philosopher Etienne Gilson in his foreword to *The Poetics of Space*, in which he suggests that Bachelard's concept of formal imagination is 'fond of novelty, picturesqueness and variety', whereas his material imagination is 'attracted to the elements of permanency present in things' (Gilson 1992, p. xiii). Although he seeks a 'dual participation' between the two, Bachelard favours the material imagination as he believes that it goes 'beyond the attraction of the imagination of forms' and derives its image from nature (Bachelard 2005, p. 31). Unlike formal imagination, which is reliant on the visual perception of images, the material imagination 'thinks matter, dreams it, lives it, or in other words materialises the imagery' (Ibid.). Applied to his re-imagining of Paris at night time, the 'concrete' noises of the city may be understood to be material sounds, while the 'abstract' sounds of the sea belong to the realm of the formal imagination.

Bachelard's belief in the significance of matter as a source of imagination is significant because it supports a type of creativity that draws on the agency of the material environment. It connects with the concept of the care collective, drawn from Latour, in which humans and 'non-humans' are equal components in relationship-centred care. The notion of a 'material imagination' offers an intriguing possibility for a creative exploration of sound, as it suggests that everyday sounds, which belong to the material world of the care home, may be understood as sensory affordances. For example, the sound of a kettle boiling or plates being washed up in the kitchen may create a 'homely' aesthetic, similar to what the sensory ethnographer Sarah Pink describes as a 'domestic soundscape' (Pink 2004, p. 72). I was interested in whether these everyday sounds could offer a sense of familiarity to the residents, in the same way that Martin Welton describes the familiarity that an actor experiences 'when sensing herself in contact with the boards of the stage' (2012, p. 124). This possibility was explored during the workshop sessions, by inviting the participants to engage closely with the everyday sounds of the room.

During a vocal warm up exercise I invited the group to close their eyes and breathe deeply, listening to the sounds of their breath and their bodies. After a few moments of breathing together I opened it out and asked everyone to listen to the sounds of the room. We listened in silence for about a minute before returning our attention to our breath. I invited the group to make a soft humming sound. Moving through different pitches, I encouraged them to explore the sensation that the vibrations made in different parts of their body, and how changes in pitch moved these vibrations into different places. This part of the exercise was important for those participants who were hard of hearing, for whom identifying the different sounds in the room may have been difficult. By exploring how sound resonated within our bodies, my intention was that the participants would be able to feel the sounds as well as hear them. For example, a high-pitched whine could be felt vibrating in the nose or the forehead, and a low throbbing hum could be felt in the chest. We then returned to listening to the sounds of the space and I invited participants to name the sounds that they could hear.

A range of different sounds were identified from inside and outside the space: the hum of the kitchen extractor fan, the sound of others breathing, the distant rumble of traffic, and a conversation in the corridor outside the room. The effect of the exercise, as well as warming up our voices for work, was that we began to explore the connection between the sounds of our bodies and the sounds of the room. By alternating our attention between our breath and the space, we were able to engage more actively with the dining room as a creative audio environment. This process included identifying what sounds we could hear but also how they travelled across different surfaces in the room, and, crucially, how we responded to them.

One woman commented on the birds that she could hear on the patio and remarked that it was a sound she had not noticed before. In this sense, the exercise broadened out the possibilities of the dining room as space which was constructed not just through 'care home sounds', but also through outdoor sounds and sounds from nature. Additionally, this process of active listening created a shared audio experience between us which in turn helped us to imagine the room as creative space. As the sound artist Brandon LaBelle remarks: 'the acoustical event is also a social one: in multiplying and expanding space, sound necessarily generates listeners and a multiplicity of acoustical 'viewpoints' adding to the acoustical event the operations of sociality … the crowd adds character to sound materially, as well as socially…' (LaBelle 2006, p. x). The idea that sounds are not only received but are also materialised through the process of collective listening supports the possibility of a dining room as an imagined space, as it draws attention to how audio environments are constructed not just through the activities of the space but through the bodies and listeners that inhabit them. This challenges the idea of a 'care home soundscape' which is a manifestation of institutional activity, and opens up the possibilities of the dining room as a creative space which is brought into being through an exchange between the sound and the listener.

In distinguishing between hearing and seeing, the philosopher Jean Luc Nancy writes about the relational character of sound. He observes that 'sound is ... made of referrals: it spreads in space where it resounds while still resounding in me' (Nancy 2007, p. 7). He also suggests that the act of listening is a key part of how a sound is created or 'made resonant': 'in the case of the ear this is a withdrawal and turning inward, a making resonant... (p. 3). This resonant relationship between sound and subject, which is understood by Nancy as something which resonates *through* bodies, and brought into being through the process of listening, offers a useful insight into the importance or listening in our project. It suggests that the participants of the sound project were active agents in the creation of the sounds that they heard. This idea is supported by the ethnomusicologist Steven Feld who suggests that 'soundscapes are perceived as and interpreted by human actors who attend to them as a way of making their place in and through the world. Soundscapes are invested with significance by those whose bodies and lives resonate with them in social time and space' (Feld 2003, p. 184).

Nancy and Feld's interpretation of listening as a type of place-making supports the relational potential of sound in a care home and the idea that the construction of a care space is a responsibility which is shared between humans and 'non-humans'. In the same way that sounds from outside the care home often evoked other times and places from the lives of the residents, the process of actively listening to the space during the warm-up exercise demonstrated the potential of sound in creating a *sense* of place. This was evident in Pauline's response to the listening exercise, in which she remarked that the noise of the extractor fan 'sounds like the machines we had in the launderette'. She then went on to say 'I used to iron Frank Sinatra's shirts you know'. The associations that Pauline made between the sound of the extractor fan, the sound of the East London launderette where she had worked as a young woman, and then her memory of ironing Frank Sinatra's shirts—whether this was true or not did not matter—illustrated the way that everyday sounds can create connections with other places and times that are significant to the lives of the residents.

The relational possibilities of sound and listening were illustrated further during a session which was dedicated to making soundscapes from everyday objects. The use of everyday objects to create musical sounds was developed primarily by the American composer John Cage in the 1950s. In *Water Walk* (1959) for example, Cage uses, among other things, the sound of ice cubes in a blender, a sauce pan lid being pushed into a bathtub of water, and five portable radios being pushed off the edge of a table onto the floor. Writing on John Cage's early work with household objects, David Dunn observed that 'through the 'musical' manipulation of the noises of everyday life, they achieved an understanding of the meaning of these sounds as an aesthetic phenomena, opportunities for a deepened awareness of the world we live in' (Dunn 2009, p. 3). Cage's dedication to the aesthetic and acoustic value of household objects inspired my decision to explore the household objects of the dining room at Mildmay. I was interested in how these ordinary objects, which belonged to the everyday world of the dining room, may be seen as creative objects in their own right, but also how they may be used to create new audio experiences within the room.

For this session we collected a selection of objects that we had found in the dining room and the adjoining kitchen. These included, much to the bemusement of the care staff, a bag of lentils, a porcelain cup, a set of keys, a paper bag and a coke can. The participants were invited to choose an object and to explore the different sounds that it made with a partner. Watching the residents carefully selecting their objects offered an interesting glimpse into the attachments and associations that some of them had with certain things. A few people wanted to have the large bunch of keys, which struck me as a significant choice, as they are objects that are associated with the domestic home but they are also associated with institutions, particularly in the context of a care home. It occurred to me that keys might be a particularly sought-after object in a care home where private space is restricted, and where locks are often associated with security and safety management.

We went round the circle and 'heard' every object individually. Some people chose to make 'big noises' with their objects and others made very small sounds, tapping the object with their fingernail or gently or rubbing it in a way that was barely audible without amplification. Elena, on the other hand, took delight in making a loud noise with her coke can, particularly when she discovered that she could make a louder sound by bashing it on the frame of the wheelchair of the person next to her. Jamie recorded each of the objects as they were played and played them back to the group, increasing the volume so that everyone could hear them. After some discussion about what the sounds reminded us of, we explored playing the objects as a group. The exercise seemed to foster at first a sense of playfulness and more gradually, a collective focus as the objects fell into a sort of rhythm. One woman said that it sounded like 'feet tapping on the dance floor'. Her suggestion led to a discussion about dancing and some members of the group talked about going dancing in South London when they were younger. Sara suggested that we use the objects to create a dance hall soundscape as a group. As the group played their objects, we encouraged them to explore other sounds that they could make with their bodies which also reminded them of a dance hall. Gradually, the sounds of clapping, talking, singing, foot-tapping and whistling were added to the soundscape. When the residents were happy with the soundscape the piece was recorded and played back in the space.

The exercise, on the one hand, was an opportunity to engage differently with the 'diegetic' sounds of the room and to explore the audio potential of everyday objects beyond their intended function. As with the vocal warm-up exercise, they also presented a connection to a different set of audio environments from outside the world of the care home. By 'manipulating' the everyday objects of the dining room into audio elements in a dancehall, we were literally re-imagining the sounds of the room as sounds from another environment. Working with sounds that already belonged to the audio world of the room reiterated the possibility of the material imagination and the care home as a creative space in its own right. It showed how care spaces are not just constructed through their physical properties but are also made up of broader network of places and environments, which can be accessed through creative practice, and through the residents' imaginations. I would like to now explore the possibility of external sound and describe how non-diegetic sounds were used to bring new audio experiences into the room.

Sounding Place

In her consideration of how sound effects are utilised across different film genres, the sound theorist Felicity Colman (2009) suggests that non-diegetic sound will often fulfil an important function beyond supporting or enhancing the fictional world of the film. This function goes beyond traditional understandings of non-diegetic sound which, according to

Marina Burke, were chiefly used to 'cover scene transitions' and to 'offer a [...] temporal support of the fictional scene' (Burke 2009, p. 67). Colman focuses on the genre of the Western Film as she believes it offers a good example of how non-diegetic sounds do not just add aural meaning to the film but also act as 'affective sonic communicators' which convey something deeper about the somatic Western experience (Ibid., p. 194). She uses the examples of gunshots and whips as sound effects which operate as part of a narrative device, but which also produce a 'range of *affective* meanings within a community's ecology' (Ibid., her emphasis). In the case of Western films these affective meanings might, she suggests, be associates with plot points such as danger and death, or themes such as wilderness and rivalry. Though thematically and conceptually very different to this study of sound in a care home, Colman's analysis of non-diegetic sound offers a useful perspective on the boundaries between internal and external sound in our project. The sounds that we brought into the care home certainly created new audio experiences in the dining room but they also stimulated connections with other spaces and times in the lives of the participants. This was apparent during the first session where we explored sounds from outside the care home.

In this session we introduced two contrasting soundscapes to the group. The first was a recording of an English countryside at summer time and the second was a soundscape of a busy international airport. The airport soundscape, which lasted for about three minutes, was composed of several different sounds including tannoy announcements, aeroplanes taking off and landing, conversations and footsteps. After playing the soundscape a couple of times, the group were invited to respond with words and phrases about what they could hear. This provoked an animated discussion among the group where they tried to pinpoint the exact location of the soundscape. As they identified the different sounds that they could hear, and what they reminded them of, I wrote down their suggestions on a large sheet of paper. This was the response:

> Want someone who knows the language.
> They said the train was departing for London.
> We're on the wrong tracks.
> Footsteps.
> The whole thing will come together.
> Sad departing.
> Footsteps.

I don't like it, it's sad.
I like a good airport.
I *love* airports.
Especially—*vroooom*—I used to fly Mosquitos.
Not those—*thwack*, the little planes.
Special relationship with planes.
We used to be told what was coming next.
Pilot and co-pilot Larry.
I don't know how I got into it.
Just one of those things.
Very interesting.

The airport soundscape had generated contrasting reactions in the group, including some unhappy associations with departures and goodbyes as one resident indicated when he said: 'I don't like it, it's sad'. It also elicited a very personal response from a resident called Kenneth who had been a pilot in the RAF during the Second World War, and told us that he had a 'special relationship with planes'. Brandon LaBelle argues that sound is unique in that it has the possibility to 'simultaneously embed us with local environments' while also 'connecting us to a broader horizon' (LaBelle 2006, p. xii). His argument helps to articulate the complex interplay between internal and external places that were evoked during the exercise. The soundscape had stimulated a positive recollection of significant places, times and events in Kenneth's life prior to living at Mildmay. It seemed to resonate with his identity as an RAF pilot and the comfort and the familiarity that he associated with the sound of aeroplanes. However, these external sounds were also part of our current sensory experience of the space we were working in. Through the process of being listened to, they were given a material presence which became embedded within the audio environment of the room.

In *Listening* Nancy argues that 'sonority is not a place where the subject comes to make himself heard … on the contrary, it is a place that becomes a subject insofar as sound resounds there' (Nancy 2007, p. 17). In other words, sound has the capacity to materialise place (or places) by virtue of the fact that it is occurring within them. Applied to this investigation of sound in a care home, this suggests that sound has the ability to create a sense of place by changing the audio construction of a particular space. Performance scholar and practitioner Deirdre Heddon furthers this idea by suggesting 'if places carry sounds than arguably sound serves to place us' (Heddon 2010, p. 36). Nancy and Heddon's remarks are significant in understanding how sound-based performance can support relational dementia care in practice. They show that sound can draw attention to the wider network of spaces that make up a care community. In the same way that care spaces can feel more familiar by the presence of domestic objects, and the opportunity to complete domestic activities, the presence of sounds from outside the care home may create a sense of familiarity for residents. The relational quality of sound was perceptible in the interplay between the external places that the soundscape evoked and the sensory experience of listening and interpreting these sounds together in the 'here and now'.

The exercise also raised a question as to how 'active' soundscapes, as opposed to soundscapes that are designed to encourage relaxation, may support a broader range of encounters with place, particularly when they are associated with specific locations. Of the sound-based work that has taken place in care homes so far, this has generally been created with therapeutic intentions in mind. For example, the multisensory therapy *Snoezelen* which is increasingly being used in dementia care settings has been designed to reduce stress and create relaxing sensory environments (see Van-Weet et al. 2006). While the therapeutic possibilities of sonic experiences such as *Snoezelen* are undoubtedly worthy of investigation, the soundscape exercise suggested that engaging with a range of audio environments might stimulate important encounters with other places, times and experiences from outside the care home. LaBelle says that 'the dislocation of ambient sound from a given location and its reproduction ... within the space of another location fuels a provocative experience; for such dislocations transform not only our spatial context and awareness of location but our perceptual and cognitive map' (LaBelle 2006, p. 237). His belief that ambient sound can provide a 'provocative experience' when played in an unfamiliar location reminds us that not all sound work in care homes has to be nostalgic or relaxing. It also has the potential to stimulate memories and facilitate journeys into other places.

Musical Sound, Sonorous Bodies

> Whether or not he is a musician, for someone who listens, the very instant a sonority, a cadence, a phrase touches him ... he is propelled into an expectation, urged towards a presentiment. (Nancy 2007, p. 66)

This chapter has focused so far on how different types of sound can support a care home as a creative space. I have used the distinctions between diegetic and non-diegetic sound to explore how everyday sounds were used to create new audio experiences in the dining room, and how external soundscapes facilitated connections to other times and places in the residents' lives. However, I have given little attention to musical sound and how this affected the space. The group's singing had an effect on the space in the way that was very different to the environmental soundscapes that we created. I would like to use some of Nancy's thoughts on musical sound and sonority to explore the effect that these melodic vocal sounds had on the space, and what music in particular may offer in supporting a care home as a relational space.

Singing was a popular activity which took place in most of the sessions, both spontaneously and as a planned activity. It was an activity that everyone in the group could join in with, regardless of their ability or access needs. When we sang together as a group, some of the residents sang or hummed along to the tune. Others who were non-verbal, or spoke very few words, nodded their heads or tapped their fingers along to the rhythm. One of the residents, John, mouthed the words to the songs silently and moved his fingers in small circles in the air as if he were conducting an orchestra. Most frequently, singing was offered spontaneously in response to something that had come up in a session. For example, when we explored the countryside soundscape in session one, someone said that they could hear a river flowing. This prompted Henry to sing the song *Old Man River* from *Showboat*, which many of the residents recognised and joined in with. Singing was also used as a warm-up at the beginning of the sessions as Jamie would play songs that the residents had told him about and this would usually lead to a group sing along. In addition to singing familiar songs that were popular with the group, we also decided to teach a new song. The piece was an old folk song called *Waly Waly*. We had intended to use the song as a vocal warm-up which would lead us into a sea-themed workshop. However, the song proved so popular that it became a regular feature of our workshops each week, and was performed in the final session.

The potential of musical sound was illustrated very clearly when we introduced the song to the group. We were not sure how they would respond to a new song and were concerned that they didn't feel under pressure to pick up the tune or remember the words. However, we were also excited at the possibility of introducing a new song and finding out where it could take us creatively. Jessie sang the whole piece through once before teaching it line by line to the group in a call and response. During the first few times, the participants' voices were barely audible, although I could see their lips moving as they followed the words on the song sheet. As the tune became more familiar, the volume started to increase very slowly and the voices became more audible in the room. When it was sung for the third time Kenneth, who had watched the group in silence the first two times, surprised everyone by joining in with a deep, strong baritone voice which resonated around the space. Though no one had heard the song before, it triggered associations with other places and some of the participants started to share personal stories about the sea. Pauline told us about travelling by boat during family holidays to Margate and Henry told us about the tropical storms he had experienced in Trinidad. Amir, who had been brought up in North India, told us he had never seen the sea until he came to England as a young man. Like the environmental soundscapes, the song had connected us to other times and place from their pasts.

Nancy's ideas on musical sound and sonority are useful in articulating what was particular about the song in terms of the affect it had on the space. In *Listening*, he distinguishes between musical sound and speech by suggesting that there are different processes involved when we listen to them. When listening to speech, he suggests, there is a necessarily a process of comprehension or sense-making involved in which the listener is required to 'strain toward a present sense beyond sound' (Nancy 2007, p. 6). He explains that the French word 'entendre' means 'to hear' but that it also translates as 'comprendre', which means 'to understand' (Ibid.). Nancy argues that the proximity between these two terms has meant that philosophical concepts of listening have 'superimposed upon listening ... or else substituted for listening, something else that may be more in the order of understanding' (Ibid., p. 1). For Nancy, this connection between hearing and understanding does not account for the meanings that are derived from listening to musical sounds that do not require listeners to comprehend a verbal meaning. He explains that the meaning derived from musical sound comes from its resonation within a 'sonorous body': 'it is from sound itself that sense is offered to auscultation' (Ibid., p. 6). He goes on to explain that sound which is musically listened to may be heard 'not as an acoustic phenomenon ... but as a resonant meaning, a meaning whose sense is supposed to be found in resonance and only resonance' (Ibid., p. 7). This concept of resonance as a source of meaning spoke to the sensations that our singing elicited in our bodies and in the space, as sounds were created, sensed, and transmitted. Like the vocal warm-up exercises we did at the beginning of each session, the density of our voices singing together with their different pitches and timbres seemed to resonate further around the room and filled the space in a way that recorded sounds did not. On several occasions when we were practicing the song, staff members and other residents would stick their head round the door to see what was happening in the room. The experience emphasised the relational possibilities of musical sound, and how it can play a key role in changing the atmosphere of the space. Nancy alludes to this possibility by describing the 'matrix-like construction of resonance' (p. 36), suggesting that musical sound has the potential to create or construct atmospheres in a way that non-musical sound may not.

What was particularly interesting about the song was how it shifted over the course of the project from being a new and unfamiliar type of sound to a routine sound in our workshops. By the end of the project, we were so familiar with it that it had almost become an ordinary sound which was 'embedded' with the other everyday sounds of the dining room. This was apparent during the final session when Elena, one of the participants with dementia, sang it quietly to herself, almost subconsciously during a tea break. This was a special moment as it indicated that Elena had memories of participating in the project over the six weeks. It also highlighted how music can support the embodied memories of people with dementia and encourage different forms of recall.

Indoor Climates

In Chap. 3, I explained how the notion of an indoor climate, as conceptualised by Martin Welton, was helpful in considering the atmospheric properties of care spaces in terms of their affordances. The weather is also something which is used by Bachelard to connect the childhood house to the outside world. In the *Poetics of Space* chapter 'House and Universe', Bachelard describes an inherent connection between the intimacy of the childhood house and the vastness of the outside world. He suggests that the sense of intimacy and comfort afforded by the house is increased in torrential weather, where 'the reminder of winter strengthens the happiness of inhabiting … we feel warm *because* it is cold outside' (Bachelard 2005, pp. 39–40, his emphasis). The pervasive presence of seasons and weather are one way that Bachelard dismisses the binary distinctions of 'outside' and 'inside', which he claims are experienced that way because of the geometric nature of a house. Instead, he suggests that the outside and the inside exist 'dialectically', continually in discourse with each other and that the weather acts as a means of increasing the sensation of intimacy inside the house. Bachelard's suggestions resonate with Welton's description of the changing atmosphere of a rehearsal space, and how these changes are registered by the performer. However, rather than considering the affective capacity of weather in terms of climatic extremes, it is the everyday-ness or mundaneness of weather, Welton argues, which creates a shared sense of place, and can help us to understand its affective potential in terms of more subtle atmospheric shifts:

> As well as those intensifications of atmosphere which seize hold of or sweep over the body, there are also those which are simply, and rather lazily there, and which, like mist, drizzle or a faint whiff of perfume, do not disrupt the flow of the mundane, but float idly by it. (Welton 2012, p. 127)

This idea of an indoor climate, which is characterised by subtle changes in atmosphere, is useful in considering the relational character of sound and space within the project. Weather was a recurring theme in our workshops, in the soundscapes that we created together, as a topic of conversation and a tangible presence in the space each week. For example, when the sun would frequently cast long rectangles of light onto the dining room floor. Over the six weeks the temperature also became milder and the daffodils bloomed outside the window. This was a big talking point for the residents and when we greeted the group each week and asked how they were, people would often talk about the change in weather. In the same way that Bachelard suggests the weather can intensify our connection with the inside, Welton suggests that the weather creates a shared sense of place as it is ever-present and an experience which is shared between humans: 'People have always talked about the weather, particularly in England and the process of feeling or imagining atmospheric conditions is a shared experience' (Welton 2012, p. 126). The process of feeling, imagining and experiencing atmospheric conditions was inherent to our use of sound, presenting itself in different ways: in our conversations about the weather, in the soundscapes we created, and when rain hammered down on the skylight during the quietest monologue.

The concept of internal weather offers something particular in understanding the relationship between sound and space in a care home. Rather than thinking about the project as an attempt to transform the audio environment of the dining room, it invites performance practitioners to engage with the aural environment of a care home in a more relational way, less in terms of a transformation of space and more in terms of a shifting climate which is a shared product of the workshops and the workshop environment. One thing that did emerge in the final week was not so much how the sound piece transformed the space, but how the 'event' of the performance changed the atmosphere of the room. It was the spaces in between and around the performance itself where these shifts were most palpable. The notion of an indoor climate raises wider questions for doing creative practice in care homes: not only as to how we cultivate different atmospheres in the room, but also how the creative context of the workshop may enable us to tap into the aesthetic potential of a space.

In considering the affective nature of sound, LaBelle suggests that it is 'intrinsically and unignorably relational. It emanates, propagates, communicates, vibrates, and agitates: it leaves a body and enters others' (LaBelle 2006, p. ix). Sound offered us a particular means of exploring the everyday creativity of a care space. On one level, it drew attention to the multitude of spaces, bodies and environments which make up, and are affected by the individual 'soundscape' of a care home. This idea is supported by the sound artist Barbara Flueckiger who also uses the concept of atmosphere to consider ambient sound as a shared product between people and their environment: 'On the one hand it is related to spatial acoustics, the materials out of which the space is composed ... and on the other to the people who use the space and their activities' (Flueckiger 2009, p. 169). On another level, sound enabled us to explore how these everyday 'domestic' spaces were shaped by external sounds, atmospheres and other places which belonged to a wider aural community. As Colman suggests, these external sounds do not just add aural meaning or context. They also teach us something about the relational nature of home in residential care.

Something that we did not have the opportunity to explore in the project was the construction of public and private spaces within the wider community of the home and what sound could offer in this context. LaBelle has written extensively on the potential of personal audio technologies to allow for the 'alternative construction and experience of a given space' (LaBelle 2011, p. 97). It would be interesting to explore how sound might be used to demark personal territories and contribute to the construction of semi-private spaces within the wider spatial context of the care home. For example, in the form of personal audio equipment such as radios, headphones and iPods. Cultivating an awareness of how care spaces are constructed through these overlapping public and private audio spaces may open up a broader set of possibilities for sound art in care homes. Specifically, how sound and music may be used to maintain personal and private spaces within the wider communal context of the care home. With these questions of personal and private space in mind, I now turn to look at taste and how it is used to negotiate space within the social environment of the care home.

References

Bachelard, G. (1992). *The Poetics of Space* (M. Jolas, Trans.). Boston: Beacon Press.

Bachelard, G. (2002). *Earth and Reveries of Will: An Essay on the Imagination of Matter* (K. Haltman, Trans.). Dallas: Dallas Institute of Humanities and Culture.

Bachelard, G. (2005). *On Poetic Imagination and Reverie* (C. Gaudin, Trans.). Putnam, CT: Spring Publications.

Bakker, R. (2003). Sensory Loss, Dementia, and Environments. *Generations: Journal of the American Society on Aging, 27*(1), 46–51.

Burke, M. (2009). The Transition to Sound. In R. Doughty, J. Eisentraut, & G. Harper (Eds.), *Sound and Music in Film and Visual Media: A Critical Overview* (pp. 58–86). New York: Continuum.

Cage, J. (1959). Water Walk. As Performed on *I've Got a Secret*, 1960. Retrieved May 21, 2014, from https://www.youtube.com/watch?v=SSulycqZH-U.

Cecire, N. (2011). Sentimental Spaces: On Mei-mei Berssenbrugge's Nest. *Jacket 2*. Retrieved August 14, 2014, from http://jacket2.org/article/sentimental-spaces.

Colman, F. (2009). The Western: Affective Sound. In R. Doughty, J. Eisentraut, & G. Harper (Eds.), *Sound and Music in Film and Visual Media: A Critical Overview* (pp. 194–207). New York: Continuum.

Dewing, J. (2009). Caring for People with Dementia: Noise and Light. *Nursing Older People, 21*, 534–548.

Dunn, D. (2009). Nature, Sound Art, and the Sacred. In D. Rothernberg & M. Ulvaeus (Eds.), *The Book of Music and Nature* (pp. 61–71). Middletown: Wesleyan University Press.

Feld, S. (2003). A Rainforest Ecoustemology. In M. Bull & L. Black (Eds.), *The Auditory Culture Reader* (pp. 223–239). Oxford and New York: Berg.

Flueckiger, B. (2009). Sound Effects: Strategies for Sound Effect in Film. In R. Doughty, J. Eisentraut, & G. Harper (Eds.), *Sound and Music in Film and Visual Media: A Critical Overview* (pp. 151–179). New York: Continuum.

Gilson, E. (1992). Foreword. In G. Bachelard, *The Poetics of Space*. (M. Jolas, Trans). Boston: Beacon Press.

Heddon, D. (2010). The Horizon of Sound Soliciting the Earwitness. *Performance Research, 15*(3), 36–42.

LaBelle, B. (2006). *Background Noise: Perspectives in Sound Art.* New York: Continuum.

LaBelle, B. (2011). *Acoustic Territories: Sound Culture and Everyday Life.* New York: Continuum.

McAvinchey, C. (2013). Coming of Age: Arts Practice with Older People in Private and Domestic Spaces. *Research in Drama Education: The Journal of Applied Theatre and Performance, 18*(4), 359–373.

Moorhouse, A. (2012). *Turning.* Digital File. Retrieved August 14, 2015, from www.aynsleymoorhouse.com.

Moorhouse, A. (2014, April 11). *Sound of Mind: A Temporal Comparison of Two Audio Art Installations that Explore Memory Loss and Identity.* Unpublished Conference Paper. 8th International Conference on Cultural Gerontology, Galway.

Nagahata, K., Fukushima, T. I., Noriko, T., & Moriyama, M. (2004). What Kinds of Soundscapes Can Elderly People with Dementia Recollect? *Noise and Health, 6*(24), 63–73.

Nancy, J. (2007). *Listening.* New York: Fordham University Press.

Pink, S. (2004). *Home Truths: Gender, Domestic Objects and Everyday Life.* Oxford: Berg.

Van-Weet, J., Jannssen, B., Van Dulmen, A., Spreeuwenberg, P., Bensing, J., & Ribbe, M. (2006). Nursing Assistants' Behaviour During Morning Care: Effects of the Implementation of Snoezelen Integrated in 24-Hour Dementia Care. *Journal of Advanced Nursing, 53*(6), 656–668.

Welton, M. (2012). *Feeling Theatre.* London: Palgrave Macmillan.

CHAPTER 6

Negotiating Space through Taste

> People seem to be curating their possessions to communicate consciously or more often unconsciously, where they want to fit in society… A childhood spent marinating in the material culture of one's class means taste is soaked right through you. (Perry 2012)

In 2012 the artist Grayson Perry made a TV series called *All in the Best Possible Taste with Grayson Perry*. In it, he explores the tastes of working class, middle class and upper class communities in three UK cities, in preparation for making a collection of tapestries about modern British taste. In each episode, Perry reflects on how the personal possessions, home environments and lifestyle practices of the people he meets are indicative of their class, and the aspirations that they have towards membership of a social group. He focuses on personal possessions and the way in which they disclose a desire to convey a particular image to other people.

Perry's interest in the origins and social function of taste across different communities raises questions about the significance of taste in a care home community. Care homes are places which typically offer residents little opportunity to display or 'curate' their personal possessions. However, my work with the residents at Mildmay suggested that taste continues to be significant in a care home, despite the restrictions that are imposed by communal and institutionalised living. In understanding how artists develop their practice around the needs of a care home, I am interested in how taste is used by residents to communicate aspects of their identity to others. How do residents express their tastes in spaces which offer them

N. Hatton, *Performance and Dementia*,
https://doi.org/10.1007/978-3-030-51077-0_6

little opportunity to display their personal possessions? And what do these expressions of taste reveal about their position within the care home community?

Taste, in its various manifestations, can be a way that residents negotiate the social environment of the care home and signal their identity to others. Unlike the communities that feature in Perry's study, a care home is a community where people from a diverse range of social and cultural backgrounds are living communally. Some residents may be unable to leave the care home, either due to ill health or mobility issues. In this situation, taste can be a significant social resource, used to negotiate group situations and identify people they would like to engage with. Participation in an arts project can create opportunities for residents to express their tastes but it can also highlight differences, particularly in relation to age, class, education and cultural background. In this second practice-based chapter about performance and the care environment, I explore the significance of taste and the ways in which it can shape participation in an arts project. I consider what the expression of taste in a creative context reveals about the way that residents position themselves in a care home community. Looking at expressions of domestic and cultural taste, this chapter addresses how they are used as social resources by residents of Mildmay as well as creating personalised and private space in the context of shared living.

A Homely Effect

I begin by considering some interior design features of care homes, and how the attempt to create a 'homely effect' can, in fact, prevent them from being experienced as homely spaces. Communal care spaces such as dining rooms and lounges are typically spaces which offer residents the least opportunity to display personal tastes, as they are designed to satisfy health and safety regulations and a restricted budget. Of the decorative and domestic items that do feature, these are usually selected to cater to the broadest of tastes. In one care home that I visited, there was a triptych of square-framed photographs in the lounge which featured large sacks of brightly coloured spices and grains. In some ways, the pictures were a refreshing contrast from the sentimental style of artwork that I had seen in other care homes, which usually consisted of watercolour paintings of landscapes and flowers. However, the photographs, which were printed onto thin paper and presented in lightweight plastic frames, had the feeling of being cheaply made and mass-produced. The subject matter of the photos was generic and reminded me of the type of images that are often sold with photo frames as an example of what could go in them.

In *Distinction*, Pierre Bourdieu describes mass-produced artwork such as this as an example of the 'popular taste'. Works that fall into this category, he suggests, are 'totally devoid of artistic ambition and pretension', and designed to obtain 'maximum effect… at a minimum cost' (Bourdieu 1984, p. 380). Art historian Monica Kjellman-Chapin extends this idea in her study of kitsch, where she suggests that mass produced artefacts and images 'contain no intrinsic content, only effect' (Kjellman-Chapin 2013, p. 35). Though also exploring the potential of kitsch as something that can produce 'trenchant social and political commentaries' (Ibid., p. 38), Kjellman-Chapin's study focuses on how artefacts which are produced to target the 'popular consumerist culture' (Ibid., p. 27) are largely perceived to be 'inauthentic' and lacking in artistic merit.

Bourdieu and Kjellman-Chapin's attention to effect and authenticity is particularly apt for the aesthetics of care homes as many of the objects seem to have been placed there with effect in mind. At the same care home, there were a small number of books and out-of-date magazines in a bookcase, which give the impression of a domestic space. However, the selection of titles and the date on the magazines made them feel less like objects you would find in a home and more like something you would see in a doctor's waiting room. Similarly, the room dividers which were used to partition the lounge area from the rest of the dining room gave the effect of a lounge space, but in reality the lounge was still visibly and audibly exposed to the 'public' sphere of the dining room. The artwork in the lounge and the token display of homely objects was illustrative of this care home's positive intention to create a homely environment and to make it a more pleasant space for residents to use. However, the effect of these objects was to emphasise the absence of personal objects and the shared ownership of the space.

Familiar Objects

Despite the lack of opportunities for residents to display their possessions in care homes, I have observed that the residents at Mildmay often appropriate objects and furniture in communal spaces as their own. One resident called Jean has scrawled her name in red marker pen across one of the dining room chairs in order to prevent anyone else from using it. The importance that she attaches to this particular chair was apparent during a film screening when she arrived late and discovered that another resident was sat in it. Visibly upset, Jean left the room and could not be persuaded to return, even when it was suggested that the other resident switch chairs. Similarly, Elena has taken a large green cushion from the lounge area—one of the only fabric cushions that I have seen at the care home. She carries the cushion around on her walking frame and uses it to reserve 'her' chair in the dining room at mealtimes, which is positioned at the far end of the room, away from the other residents. The care staff told me that she prefers to dine on her own and that the cushion enables her to maintain a space at her chosen table.

The gerontologists Jill Harrison and John Ryan suggest that attachments to objects in later life may be 'analogous to the shedding and storing of personal possessions' (Harrison and Ryan 2010, p. 650), implying that opportunities to express taste become much more significant when personal possessions are reduced. This suggests that the appropriation of communal objects at Mildmay may be a response to a reduction in personal possessions. Personalising objects that belong to the care home, through appropriation or by mark-making, may be a strategy for residents to create personal space in communal areas. Bourdieu argues that certain types of taste are 'born out of necessity', and that particular circumstances impose 'a taste for… and consequently acceptance of the necessary, a resignation to the inevitable' (Bourdieu 1984, p. 373). This idea is applicable to the appropriation of everyday objects in communal care spaces, as residents may be adjusting to a reduction in their own possessions. The fact that the residents at Mildmay are unable to display their own homely objects in the lounge may have led to them forming attachments to the objects that are available in the room. The objects that Elena and Jean selected were unremarkable; there was nothing that made Jean's chair stand out from the other armchairs in the room. However, assuming ownership of these objects enabled these women to literally carve out personal space within the communal context of the dining room.

In *Subculture: The Meaning of Style*, the sociologist Dick Hebdige describes how objects, particularly domestic objects, are appropriated and to used 'express certain meanings' within a particular group (Hebdige 1979, p. 18). Using the example of the safety pin as a domestic object that was re-appropriated by punks as a statement of subversion and rebellion, Hebdige argues that 'humble objects can be magically appropriated: 'stolen' by appropriate groups and made to carry secret meanings: meanings which express, in code, a form of resistance to the order which guarantees their continued subordination' (Ibid.). The iconic image of the Punk safety pin does not seem immediately comparable to 85-year-old Elena carrying around a cushion on her walking frame. However, her behaviour could be interpreted as a form of resistance to the regulations of a care space. Elena's decision to take the cushion involved a process of appropriation which was attached to a rebellious act: the decision to dine on her own at a table away from other residents. Similarly, Jean's decision to scrawl 'JEAN' in several places across the dining room chair is an act which would be deemed anarchic in other contexts and is a statement of ownership in an environment where little is owned or chosen by residents themselves.

Bourdieu's work on objects and capital offers a useful perspective on how the appropriation of ordinary objects in a care home may afford residents a particular status within the care home community. In *Distinction* he suggests that 'social relations are objectified within things', and that the daily contact people have with 'familiar, intimate objects which are there' reveal a certain type of taste (Bourdieu 1984, p. 70). He develops this idea in *The Form of Capital* where he uses the term 'objectified cultural capital' to describe how status is achieved and transmitted through material objects: 'The cultural capital objectified in material objects and media, such as writing, painting, monuments, instruments etc, is transmissible in its materiality' (Bourdieu 1986, p. 50). Though the objects that Bourdieu are describing are objects associated with arts and culture, he also suggests that 'social relations' are present in all sorts of objects, which 'in their luxury or poverty, their distinction or vulgarity, their 'beauty' or 'ugliness' impress themselves through bodily experiences' (Bourdieu 1984, p. 70).

In addition to revealing the tensions that exist between the residents and the care home, the appropriation of everyday objects at Mildmay may also indicate the power dynamics that exist between residents in the battle to carry out personal routines. Jean has ensured that no one else can use her armchair or she will refuse to take part in social activities. Similarly, Elena's opportunity to dine alone affords her a status among other residents, as the opportunities to have private space outside of their rooms are limited.

Coincidently, Bourdieu's description of the sensory qualities of everyday objects evokes many of the sensory properties of care homes. In describing the unconscious process in which objects acquire social relations, he writes of the 'quiet caress of beige carpets or the thin clamminess of tattered, garish linoleum, the harsh smell of bleach or perfume as imperceptible as a negative scent' (Ibid., p. 70). This description suggests that expressions of personal taste are not wholly removed from the sensory experience of taste. In addition to being something which is cultivated though education and upbringing, the process of acquiring taste is very much an embodied one which stems from responses to colour, texture, smell and other sensory properties. Bourdieu's attention to how taste is manifest and experienced through 'bodily experiences' (an idea which he develops further in his concept of 'habitus'), raises interesting questions for people living with dementia. Both Jean and Elena have dementia and Marian, the activity coordinator, explained to me that since Jean's diagnosis (which happened after she had moved to Mildmay) she had become 'very particular' about her routine. In addition to using her chair, I noticed that at mealtimes she would use the same plastic water glass with purple flowers on it and the same table mat. It is possible that the decision to appropriate objects may also be attributable to dementia and the need that these residents have to find familiar objects in an unfamiliar environment.

The attachment that these residents showed to ordinary domestic objects raises questions about the potential of creative practice in supporting residents with dementia to engage with familiar objects. Arts practices in care homes can broaden the material experience of the care home by introducing new objects. This in turn can yield insights into residents' tastes, as well as highlighting the possibilities of introducing objects from outside the world of the care home. Reflecting on her experience of doing a performance with drama students at a care home, Helen Nicholson described a moment where one of the residents started to collect up the props that had been used in the performance. Citing Kitwood, she explains that the moment marked a turning point in their work as they realised that 'hiding and losing objects may be part of a person's attempt to 'make things safe' when there is an overpowering sense that things are continually being taken away' (Nicholson 2011, p. 52). They realised that offering the resident objects to touch, only to remove them later 'exacerbated her anxiety' and that if they gave her objects to keep 'she became calmer and increasingly able to participate in the activities' (Ibid.).

Kitwood's idea that retaining objects can be a way for people with dementia to 'keep things safe' may be also interpreted as a practice of 'care work' when considered in terms of the attention that these residents gave to their chosen objects. The term 'care work' is used by the anthropologist Daniel Miller in his book *The Comfort of Things*, which examines the lifestyle practices of different households on a South London street. Miller uses the term 'care work' to describe how the care and attention that individuals give to domestic objects in their environment is comparable to the care that they give to the people around them. This is an idea which is central to the relational framework for dementia care and the notion that people with dementia are equal contributors to the caregiving relationship. As an arts practitioner, I am interested in the opportunities that domestic objects provide for residents to engage in caring practices and how participation in arts workshops may support these opportunities.

Objects and Care Work

Shortly after the sound project had finished at Mildmay, I was invited to run a workshop with residents in order to consult them about the re-design of a space at the home. The decision to re-design the reception area came from an acknowledgement that a group of residents with dementia preferred to use it as a social space to the lounge. Marian explained to me that they liked to sit there because they could see the comings and goings of the care home. It was a busy thoroughfare between different parts of the building and the seating area was arranged as such so that they could see the entrance to the care home as well as the corridor which ran between the dining room and the residents' bedrooms. The idea was to make the reception into a more pleasant and homely space for these residents to sit in.

For the workshop I brought in a selection of objects and materials. Some of these materials were associated with decorating, such as wallpaper samples, home magazines, paint charts and fabrics of different colours and textures. I also brought a selection of natural and scented objects including wood, candles, soaps and some images of places that the residents had told me they liked to visit. A washing line was strung across the space to hold the larger pieces of fabric and to draw attention to any images that the participants liked. Residents were invited to create mood boards by ripping out images and sticking them with masking tape to a large piece of cardboard. For the residents whose hands were unsteady, care staff helped them to cut out and stick their images to their board.

I had explained to the residents that mood boards were 'supposed to be rough' and encouraged them to rip the images they liked from the home magazines without worrying about being neat. However, each of the participants approached this task with great care and attention. Some of them were concerned about ripping samples from the sheets of wallpaper because they didn't want to ruin them. The attention that Lydia gave to her mood board was particularly interesting. Her process of choosing images was slow and methodical, as she carefully selected photographs from different magazines, making sure that the colours matched. I watched as she cut out a photograph of a vase of flowers extremely slowly, taking particular care with the edges. After she had cut out her images she placed them out in front of her and spent a good deal of time arranging and rearranging them on the board before she stuck them down neatly. Not every image that she had cut out of the magazines made the final mood board and when she had finished she asked me for an envelope to keep the spare pictures in, telling me that she was going to keep them for her scrap book. Her final mood board consisted of a small selection of coordinated images associated with country homes: grand looking red brick houses set in grounds and lots of garden images such as seeds, bulbs and flowers Fig. 6.1.

In *The Comfort of Things*, Daniel Miller explores some of the different ways that people attend to objects in their home environments. He suggests that the relationships people have with their possessions often represent integral aspects of their relationships with people. Challenging the subject-object dichotomy, he suggests that people can become objects of care in the same way that objects can become subjects of relationships. The focus of his enquiry is on possessions which do not necessarily have financial value but which have a particular value to their owners because they symbolise a specific type of knowledge, an investment of time, or family history. He uses the example of a man caring for his stamp collection as something which also illustrates his caring disposition towards people:

> The connection between the way he cares for stamps… and the way he cares for people throughout his life is not just one of analogy. Both activities are properly described as care work in the broadest sense because they are both saturated with moral principles—which, if anything, are more explicit in the relation to objects. (Miller 2009, p. 26)

Miller's interest in how individuals demonstrate 'care work' in their home environments suggests that certain objects in care homes may support caregiving behaviour among residents, particularly for those living with dementia. The seriousness with which the residents approached the task of creating their mood boards and the care that they took in selecting the 'right' images demonstrated the reciprocal potential of the caregiving

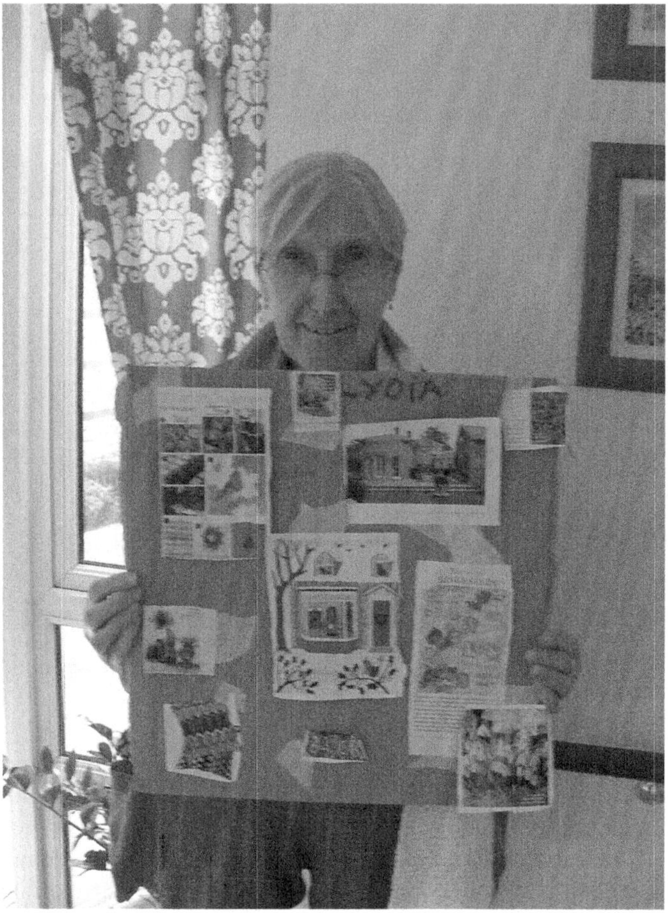

Fig. 6.1 Mildmay resident Lydia with her mood board, 2014. (Photograph by Nicky Hatton)

relationship. Interestingly, many of the samples that the residents chose matched their own clothing. For example, Rose's mood board was a wash of subtle pinks and purples which matched her cardigan and her nail varnish. Her nails were long and immaculately shaped and each week that I came to the care home they were painted a different colour. The attention that she paid to maintaining her physical appearance was a practice of care

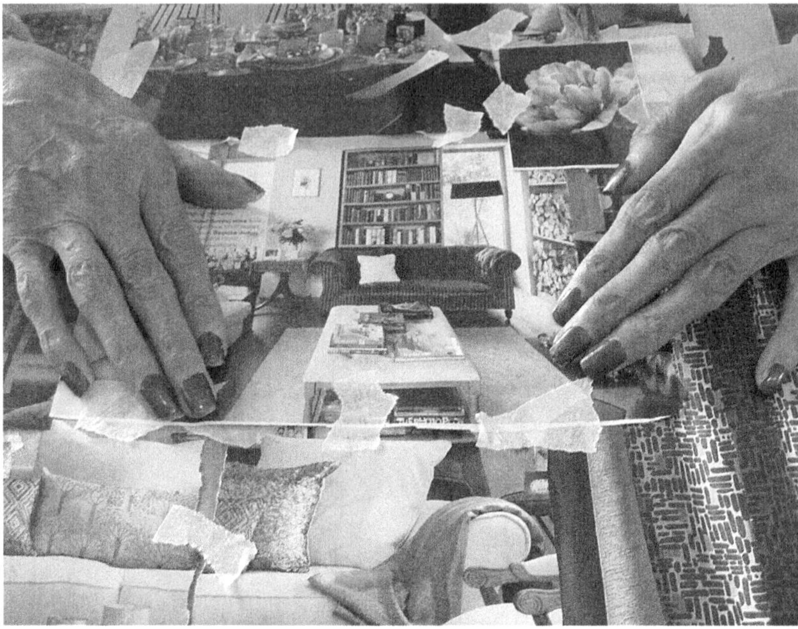

Fig. 6.2 Mildmay resident Rose with her nail varnish matching her mood board, 2014. (Photograph by Nicky Hatton)

work in itself and drew attention to the significance of dress as an embodied expression of taste in a care home (Fig. 6.2).

The sociologists Julia Twigg and Christina Buse reflect on the significance of clothing and dress for people with dementia. Drawing on Pia Kontos' study of embodied selfhood, they argue that clothing is an embodied aspect of social identity and that the 'material, tactile aspects of clothing' can remain particularly important (Twigg and Buse 2013, p. 329). They hint at the social significance of dress for people with dementia, arguing that 'clothes lie at the interface between the body and its social presentation.... signify[ing] to the wider world who and what the person is' (Ibid., p. 327). Similarly, in her investigation of how selfhood is expressed at a pre-reflective level, Pia Kontos reflected on how the tastes and class values of the residents were expressed in relation to clothing, using the example of a woman who would 'reach behind her neck to pull from beneath her bib a string of pearls she wore so that they could be seen' (Kontos 2005, p. 561). Their studies resonate with my own work, as many of the social interactions I had with the female residents at Mildmay were about clothing. For example, one resident would frequently ask me where I bought my skirt, and I would compliment her in turn on her jewellery. However, while these studies hint at the social significance of taste, they do not consider how taste contributes to social networks within the care home. Furthermore, while their attention to how social values are expressed through clothing and jewellery is relevant to the female residents, it does not necessarily account for the male residents, whose tastes were expressed in different ways.

In my experience of running arts projects in care homes, I have often found it difficult to engage male residents. This challenge is well documented by charities such as Age UK, who have developed projects with the specific aim of engaging men in sociable activities.[1] The challenge is exacerbated by the fact that the majority of care work is undertaken by women. As Mary Daly and Katherine Rake remark in their study of gender and the welfare state, 'one of the seeming constants across [European] nations is a feminization of the caring sector. As the sector has grown, women have formed an even larger majority of paid care workers' (Daly and Rake 2003, p. 56). The low representation of men within the care sector means that it can be harder to know what type of activities male residents will enjoy. The complex relationship between gender, participation and taste was particularly apparent during the film and music project, which I now turn to.

Taste beyond Nostalgia

There has been little research on cultural taste in later life, particularly in the context of residential care. This is starting to be explored by gerontologists who are interested in the cultural dimension of ageing. I begin with an idea that has been advanced by the gerontologists Murray Forman and Andy Bennett: that musical taste is significant to how people express their identities in later life. The wellbeing benefits of music in care homes has been considered extensively in recent years, but the significance of musical taste has not been explored. As Bennett and Taylor suggest, this literature fails to discuss 'the specificities of musical taste, genre and what forms of popular music ageing subjects use' (Bennett and Taylor 2012, p. 233). Rather than associating musical consumption with reminiscence, which is the focus of many musical studies in care homes, Bennett argues that 'ageing audiences for popular music often exhibit a dynamic, shifting and developing quality in the appreciation of music, its relevance to their everyday lives and its broader sociocultural significance' (Bennett 2013, p. 2).

The majority of Bennett's field work involves conducting research with music fans who are approaching middle age, rather than people who have actually reached old age, although some of Bennett's research participants joked that they would 'still be listening to the Ramones in the old people's home' (2013, p. 179). However, his focus on the dynamic and aesthetic nature of taste patterns in later life is relevant to how people in care homes use taste to construct their identities in an ongoing fashion. Furthermore, his study raises an important question as to how the tastes of the care home population are evolving with each generation—something that is discussed later in this chapter. In this section, I attempt to unpick the sociocultural significance of musical taste in residential care. I suggest that looking beyond music as a form of reminiscence or nostalgia can foster understandings of how musical taste is an important and current aspect of an older person's identity. Rather than focusing on the nostalgic or reminiscence qualities of listening to music in care homes, this part of the chapter is concerned with how musical taste is used by residents as an *ongoing* articulation of their identity as they negotiate the social environment of the care home. In order to do this, I must first explore some of the assumptions and stereotypes attached to musical taste in old age. Some of these assumptions have been identified by Bennett and Forman and some I have observed from my own work in care homes.

A common assumption I have encountered in care homes is that the residents will enjoy the music that was most popular when they were teenagers and young adults. For many of the residents who were born in the 1920s and 1930s, Frank Sinatra is a familiar musical icon and one which appears very frequently. I have encountered Frank Sinatra in care homes and day centres in the UK and North America in activity spaces, lounges dining rooms and residents' bedrooms. While the popularity of Sinatra among some members of this age group is evident, his prevalence at care homes does not account for the diversity of musical tastes that exist with a care home community, and differences in age, gender, cultural and social background. Furthermore, it points to an assumption that older people must 'almost by necessity, like old music, music from their youthful years' (Forman 2012, p. 246).

Forman challenges the widely accepted assumption that 'in their advanced years people tend to disengage from popular culture, losing their connection with evolving trends and tastes and gradually becoming isolated' (Ibid.). He argues that an acceptance that older people will naturally disengage from popular culture as their personal networks shrink reinforces 'social labelling and ageist perspectives... that tend to de-legitimise the musical tastes of older citizens' (Ibid., p. 245). Drawing on his own observations of popular music programmes in American care homes, he explains that many activity coordinators who are responsible for programming musical activities for residents will adopt a sentiment of 'music you can understand'—a tagline used by a National radio station in America to attract older listeners. Accompanying this perception, he suggests, is an assumption that listening to this music involves a sort of 'nostalgically yearning' for better times. Forman argues that the 'effect can be corrosive, as the elder subject is effectively displaced from present-day sensibilities and dislocated from contemporary cultural forms or practices' (Ibid., p. 246).

As an alternative, Forman attempts to identify what these tastes cultivated in youth may offer an older person as they negotiate their identities in later life. He suggests that recalling the music of the past doesn't necessarily suggest a desire to return to that period of life. Rather, expressing musical tastes that were developed in their youth may be a way that older people engage with, or make sense of, their present circumstances. He illustrates this idea by drawing on the historian Kimberley Smith's concept of nostalgia.

Smith traces the historical lineage of the term 'nostalgia', arguing that rather than a wistful longing for times past, being nostalgic can be a way of organising feelings about the present. She explains that nostalgia is 'not just a name attached to a universal, brute feeling, but a particular way of ordering and interpreting the various ideas, feelings and associations we experience when thinking of the past. To experience a memory nostalgically is not just to have certain feelings along with that memory but to adopt a particular attitude towards it' (Smith 2000, p. 509). Her view is echoed by Grayson Perry who describes nostalgia as 'the emotional structures that formed the taste' (Perry 2012), implying that nostalgia has a practical function in how people develop and express their tastes. Smith rightfully suggests that remembering positive aspects of the past 'does not necessarily indicate a desire to return there. Remembering the past should instead be seen as a way to express valid desires and concerns about the present' (Smith 2000, p. 523).

This concept of nostalgia is particularly valuable as it suggests that the musical tastes that care home residents had in their youth are a meaningful aspect of how they negotiate their identity in the present. This idea is endorsed by Andy Bennett and Jodie Taylor who suggests that musical taste is a 'cultural resource' which people use to negotiate their identities in later life. Challenging what they consider to be a sociological preoccupation with music and youth culture, they suggest that popular music retains a 'critical currency for ageing audiences as a key operative modality of identity, lifestyle and associated cultural practices' (Bennett and Taylor 2012, p. 232). They suggest that 'ageing identities and lifestyles are also reflexive constructs that draw on and symbolically transform available images, objects and texts, including music' (Ibid., p. 236). Their argument that music is a tool that can be drawn on in the construction of ageing identity is pertinent to how cultural taste is used to communicate or conceal certain aspects of the self to other residents in a care home. This idea can be understood further with an example from Mildmay.

Henry is a man in his early 80s who has dementia. He was born in Trinidad in the 1930s and spent some time attending school there as a child before moving to England in his early teens to attend a private boys' school. Henry enjoys talking about his school days and often told me about the English poetry that was drummed into him at school. He has a good singing voice and regularly seized upon opportunities to entertain with the poetry and songs he used to sing when he was younger. Given the opportunity, Henry would sing the song *Too Young* by Nat King Cole. His performance was usually introduced with an explanation that he was 'gifted with a good singing voice' and that at school he was frequently encouraged to perform. Each time Henry sang, he received enthusiastic applause from care staff and other residents, which seemed to please him.

Henry's recitals at the care home were inspired by a habit from his past; the routine of performing to his peers at school and on social occasions. However, rather than his singing being a nostalgic remnant of his past, or a symptom of Henry's dementia leaving him 'stuck in the past', his singing enabled him to communicate aspects of his identity to others. The act of singing established him as talented performer and the anecdote about attending boys' school in England established him as someone who had achieved a private education at a prestigious school. Additionally, the frequency of his recitals revealed something about his social position at Mildmay; that he was used to having an audience. His accustomedness to performing and receiving praise from other residents positioned him as a dominant figure within the care home. Though they were wonderful to listen to, Henry's recitals would often dominate the sessions as we had to wait until he had finished singing before we could move on. Henry's weekly performances hinted towards the power dynamics that exist within a care home community and how these can be revealed or even amplified though participation in an arts project. It was an indication that while group arts practices in care homes can enable some residents to express aspects of their identity, they can simultaneously restrict others from doing so.

Negotiating the diverse tastes of the residents in a group arts project can be challenging, particularly as the opportunities that residents have to express their tastes are usually limited. However, it can also reveal the potential of taste as a social tool within the care home. For the remainder of this chapter, I consider the social implications of taste and how the nature of participation in an arts workshop reflects the social dynamic of the home. This will be explored in relation to a film and popular music project that I facilitated at Mildmay over a three-month period. I have chosen to focus on musical taste because music was the most popular art form in the project but it was also at times a source of tension and disagreement between residents.

Taste and Social Networks

In *Out of Time*, a book that explores the 'perils and pleasures of ageing', Lynne Segal suggests that friends become harder to find in old age, particularly when 'our elective affinities may reside with communities that have faded away' (Segal 2014, p. 255). Her perspective is shared by Harrison and Ryan who point out that opportunities for older people to retain social networks in later life are often restricted by 'functional, physical and structural limitations, such as institutionalisation, lack of transport and disability' (Harrison and Ryan 2010, p. 652). They argue that this issue is particularly critical for people in care homes who, in addition to leaving their homes, often have to leave an old neighbourhood as well. In acclimatising to this loss, care home residents are also required to adjust to being part of a new community. Those who are unable to leave the care home independently are likely to encounter the same people repeatedly in communal spaces and must make choices about how they engage with the social life of the home, as well as finding strategies for negotiating personal space.

Ryan and Harrison suggest that under these circumstances, taste can be a 'relational tool' used to navigate the social environment of the care homes and facilitate social interactions with others (Ibid., p. 649). Drawing on the sociologist Paul DiMaggio's work, they argue that musical taste in particular can 'provide fodder for least-common denominator talk and gives strangers something to talk about, facilitating the sociable intercourse necessary for acquaintances to ripen into friendships' (1987, p. 443). Their argument draws attention to the social value of taste in care homes and how this might be supported through participation in an arts project. Group arts projects can increase the opportunities for residents to come together in a social setting, as well as offering them the chance to engage with different cultural forms. The film and music club brought together residents from two different sites who would not normally have socialised together, except during parties and special occasions. Moreover, the familiarity of the popular music and films that were played during these sessions provided these residents with conversational 'fodder'. However, though Ryan and Harrison argue that music is an important social resource, they do not account for is why music might be an effective form of social capital, or whether different types of musical taste provide different degrees of social capital for older people. These questions are addressed in this chapter.

Coincidentally, the film and music club originated from my interest in the care home reception area as a social space. Following the interior design session, I had been considering how I might introduce creative activities that could support the residents to use it as social space. My intention had been to hold weekly film screenings that were themed around places that the residents liked to visit. In the week following the design session, I sourced a projector and prepared a selection of film footage of seaside towns, gardens and other places that they had told me about. However, two things happened which meant I had to change my plans. In the days leading up to the first screening the care home manager said that we could not use the reception area for activities as she was concerned that it posed a health and safety hazard. Consequently, the workshop had to be moved to the staff meeting room down the corridor. The second change happened when I came to drop the projector off and test the equipment in the space. As I set up the projector some of the residents approached me to find out what I was doing. When I explained about the film screenings that started to talk about the film stars and musicians that they liked. As a result, I began to source a collection of clips based on the music and films they had told me about.

The 'Old Film and Music Club', as it was named by Marian, was the most well-attended project that I had been involved in at Mildmay with an average of 12 residents attending each week. As the screenings were taking place in a room off a corridor, many residents would often find out about it as they were walking past and would decide to join in. After the first three weeks of running the sessions in the meeting room we had to move the project into the dining room in order to fit everyone's wheelchairs in. Sessions were between an hour and 90 minutes long, depending on the participants' concentration and involved, quite simply, watching film clips together on a big screen and discussing them over tea and cake. The content of the workshops varied each week and I attempted to theme the sessions, while also including a variety of music and films that reflected the broad tastes of the residents. By the end of the project I had several hours of film footage; a selection of live music performances from the 1940s, 1950s and 1960s, musicals, films and sketches, based on what the residents had told me about. A reflective account of a particular workshop gives an idea of the diversity of tastes that existed among the participants. This workshop also illustrated the social relationships that existed between members of the group and how these were played out through space.

> It is a Tuesday afternoon in August and I have arrived to run a session in the dining room. The room is muggy and airless and the mood slightly fractious. Since the project has moved to the dining room, I have stopped using the projector as the space is much larger and some of the residents cannot hear the sound when it is played through portable speakers. A few residents have gathered by the time I arrive and watch expectantly as I fiddle with cables, trying to get my laptop to speak to the large flat screen television. I have spent the weekend sourcing a collection of clips based on conversations from last week. These include 50s and 60s pop music, and a broad selection of film clips. Rose yells sharply as the TV screen flickers and switches from a quiz show to my computer desktop. I can't fully make out her words but I think she's saying 'You broke it, you broke it'. I apologise awkwardly and ask her if she would like to see some Charlie Chaplin, who she enjoyed the previous week. 'No', she states emphatically, and turns her head away from me. I plough on nervously and begin with a clip of '60s heartthrob Adam Faith performing to a crowd of hysterical teenagers. Ida springs into life, singing and moving her arms around, blowing extravagant kisses at the screen. Shirley, who is sat next to her, laughs and sings along, moving her

> arms in sync. Elena enters the room with her green cushion balanced carefully on her walker and makes a slow and determined beeline for the sofa where Dora is sat. I offer to place her cushion on the sofa for her. Dora shakes her head at me and mouths 'no'. As Elena sits, she leans her body as far away from her as possible for the duration of the session. David listens quietly and attentively to the music until the clip has finished and then politely asks me if I've 'got any Marlon Brando'. As I root through my iTunes for the scene from *On the Waterfront* where Charley tries to convince Terry not to testify, Pauline pipes up from the back of the room and says she would prefer to see *Random Harvest*. She is sat at her own table on her own, a safe distance from the 'hub' of the group. Elena glares at her and mutters furiously under her breath. Amir hangs back shyly in the doorway, leaning on his crutches.

This session demonstrated one of the biggest challenges of the project, which was trying to accommodate the diverse tastes of the residents. The resolution with which some of the participants vocalised their choices for different types of film and music and the disagreements that arose between them reflected the diversity of tastes, and perhaps the lack of opportunities that they had to engage with the popular culture they had enjoyed before they moved to the care home. The session also illustrated some of the tensions that can arise from group-based projects. Though each of the residents had chosen to attend the group, it was apparent that several of them did not get along with each other. What interested me about this session was how the social position of the residents seemed to be reflected spatially. Dora, for example, would always seek a 'front row' seat where she could make her suggestions heard. Amir would always stand or sit at the back of the room. As I got to know him, I realised that he liked to keep himself to himself and would rarely take part in activities which involved him interacting with the other residents.

In his concept of social capital, Bourdieu used the concept of homophily to suggest that people are more likely to associate with those who are socially similar to themselves: 'the exchanges instituting mutual acknowledgement presuppose the re-acknowledgement of objective homogeneity' (Bourdieu 1986, p. 51). In other words, social relationships are cultivated through recognition of similarities in taste. He describes social capital as '…a durable network of more or less institutional relationships of mutual acquaintance and recognition… which provides each of its members with the backing of the collectively owned capital, a credential which entitles them to credit in the various sense of the word' (Ibid.). Following

Bourdieu, music might be understood as a type of 'social capital' in a care home, used by residents to identify people who have similar interests to them and support social interactions. Pop music was the most popular type of music among the residents, particularly for those who had been teenagers in the 1950s when pop music was emerging as a genre in Britain and North America. The mutual appreciation of musicians such as Bill Hayley, Elvis and the Beatles led to conversations between those who had enjoyed listening to them when they were younger. On occasions, similarities in musical taste were related to the social and geographical backgrounds of the residents. Ida and Shirley were both born in East London and had lived there all their lives. They were of a similar age and had both been young mothers in London when Adam Faith was at the height of his success in the 1960s. This discovery seemed to foster a social connection between them as I noticed at the next session they were sat together and chose to do so for the rest of the project. The 'credit' afforded to the two women through their shared love of Adam Faith was reflected by their decision to sit together in subsequent sessions. Interestingly, both Ida and Shirley had dementia and though their musical taste was connected to their youth, the realisation that they both liked Adam Faith was something they could respond to and be conversant about 'in the moment'. The social potential of music was also reflected in the interactions that took place between other residents in the group. For example, Pauline and Jean would usually choose to sit at separate tables a little way away from the hub of the group. However, as the weeks progressed and it became apparent that they were both very knowledgeable about film musicals, I observed that they had started to sit at the same table, still a safe distance apart but close enough for them to converse about what they were watching.

Bourdieu suggests that the unconscious aim behind social capital is to establish social relationships which are 'directly usable in the short or long term, i.e., at transforming contingent relations such as those of the neighbourhood.... into relationships that are once necessary and elective' (Ibid., p. 52). In one sense, it could be argued that the mutual appreciation of music was born out of the necessity of being in social contact with other residents, and that it afforded the residents a social tool which was directly usable in the short term. However, popular music was not enjoyed by all residents and the limitations of music as a form of social capital was apparent when I consider those residents who did not enjoy it or were unfamiliar with it. One of the participants, John, was avid fan of jazz music, and he would talk knowledgeably about it whenever we played artists such as John Coltrane and Miles Davis. However, he would quickly lose interest when other music was played and found it difficult to join in with conversations about mainstream music. After the second session he did not return and I could not persuade him to come back. Marian told me that John had achieved what she described as 'a high level of education' and that he often found the activities on offer at the care home a little 'low brow'. In considering how cultural tastes develop Bourdieu suggests that the process of acquiring cultural capital is one of accumulation or 'self-cultivation': '[one which] presupposes a process of embodiment, incorporation… time which must be invested personally by the investor' (Ibid., p. 48). In some ways, John's love of jazz music set him apart from the other residents as it implied a deeper understanding of musical form, and perhaps a personal investment in the form of education or time. However, rather than increasing John's social status, the cultural capital that came with his love of jazz was a source of tension, which highlighted the differences between him and other residents, and prevented him from accessing the social capital that came from a shared appreciation of pop music. Similarly, Amir, who was born in India and hadn't moved to London until the 1970s was largely unfamiliar with British and American popular music from the 1950s and 60s. He was shy by nature and initially very reticent to talk about the music he enjoyed. I could understand his apprehension as when I eventually did play some bhangra music, another resident was critical about it.

In her book *Class, Self, Culture*, the sociologist Beverley Skeggs suggests that 'some forms of culture are condensed and inscribed onto social groups and bodies that then mark them and restrict their movement in social space, whilst others are not, but are able to become mobile and flexible' (Skeggs 2006, p. 2). Amir's taste for bhangra music, which he revealed quietly at the end of one session, restricted his participation in social aspects of the group, as it was not considered to be as socially acceptable as Western popular music. For the residents who had been brought up in the UK, the shared recognition and appreciation of popular music was a social tool which enabled them to become mobile but for Amir his musical taste served to highlight his cultural difference to the residents who had been born in Britain. His reluctance to share the music he enjoyed seemed to reflect the way that he positioned himself within the care home as each week he chose to sit outside of the circle, a little way back from the rest of the group. Amir's taste for bhangra music 'marked' him as different from the other residents and restricted his ability to engage with the social hub of the group. However, one thing I learnt about musical taste from the project is that it isn't simply *attributable* to gender, social and cultural background, or at least that the development or accumulation of taste involves a more complex process. Henry, the resident from Trinidad, had little interest in Trinidadian music and but was very vocal about his passion for English poetry and classical music. He challenged the assumption that people's tastes are necessarily rooted in their cultural or social backgrounds. Additionally, the fact he had acquired a taste for classical music in later life raised questions as to how tastes develop across the life course. If personal tastes can change in our youth is there any reason to suggest that they can't develop in later life? Although the majority of the music that the residents requested was the music they had listened to when they were younger, this does not mean that they would not enjoy music from another era. Matt Cornell (2012) hints at the possibility of this in his research into an intergenerational arts project at a care home which involved both DJ technology and old records. Cornell rightfully suggests that there is further scope to investigate the relationship between new cultural experiences and taste patterns in later life, reiterating that the development and articulation of taste in later life is a complex process which can be motivated by several factors. Furthermore, Henry's taste for classical music, developed in later life, is a good example of how the identities of people with dementia are not fixed, but are evolving and relational.

The sociologist Wendy Bottero criticises Bourdieu's reliance on homophily, arguing that 'a community of shared dispositions cannot be assumed' (Bottero 2009, p. 404). Her argument is particularly pertinent to a care home community as it is made up a diverse group of people who have not necessarily chosen to live in close proximity. The likelihood of residents associating with each other in a social situation is increased not just by commonalities but through the necessity of encountering each other on a daily basis. Bottero draws attention to the interactional properties of the space itself, claiming that 'greater attention must be paid to the substance and patterning of social networks' (Ibid.). This is a view echoed by Skeggs, who suggests that it not the object of exchange but the *nature* of the exchange itself which establishes value and meaning' (Skeggs 2006, p. 9). Their suggestions highlight the complex relationship between tastes and social networks. The social exchanges that took place between the residents at Mildmay were also influenced by the spatial dynamics of the room and the pre-existing social relationships of the care home. As the anecdote from the workshop suggests, there was no love lost between Elena and Dora, but Elena still chose to sit next to her, not because she wanted to socialise with her but because she wanted a seat on a sofa instead of a hard-backed chair. Similarly, Ida and Shirley's decision to sit together may have been motivated by the need to construct an immediate, short-term social connection. Bottero's attention to the nature of social exchange suggests that social networks in a care home can be as much to do with necessity, and a response to what is happening in the space at the time, as a desire for long-term friendship.

Positive Divergence

> As I've got older I believe less and less in the language of the independent self… [in every sense] we are never self-sustaining but constituted by others who are different from us. Another aspect of this is that I've lived between 'home', where I can't be home, and that place where I 'feel at home' but which will never be quite home. So I've learned not to mourn but to embrace displacement as a strategy for survival. (Hall in Segal 2014, p. 276)

This quotation comes from an interview that Lynne Segal conducted with Stuart Hall, not long before he died in 2014. It stood out to me because Hall is talking at the end of his life about home and how it is constituted by people, rather than a fixed place. This idea resonates with my interest in the relational qualities of a care home community. For residents, accepting the ambiguous status of a care home as a place which 'will never quite be home', and which is constituted by 'others who are different' may be a strategy for survival. What also stands out, is Hall's emphasis on difference. The diversity of tastes discussed in this chapter may be equally as important as commonalities when forming social networks in a care home.

In a study which explores divergence and taste, Jonah Berger and colleagues suggest that 'people diverge to signal their identity to others so that they can enjoy more fulfilling social interactions' (Berger et al. 2007, p. 2). Following Bourdieu, they acknowledge that taste can gain value through associations with others but argue that these tastes become diluted when 'members of more than one type hold them' (Ibid.). Grayson Perry describes this as 'the vanity of small differences' (Perry 2012), suggesting that an individual's taste is often shaped or defined by its distance from the tastes of others. However, rather than considering divergences in taste as a barrier to social interaction, Berger argues that articulating such differences can 'help achieve a healthy balance between needs for inclusion and for differentiation' in different social groups (Berger et al. 2007, p. 5).

If I reflect on the way that taste that was expressed during the film and music project, there were several occasions where differences in musical taste led to disagreements. Though these disagreements were occasionally a source of tension, they were usually good natured and often prompted social interactions. Frequently, a conversation between participants would start from a mutual dislike of an artist, or what I would describe as a 'healthy disagreement' about a song that was being played. Some residents appeared to relish the opportunity to criticise a particular artist or song. For example, when I played Cliff Richard, who was popular with several older members of the group, Ida, who was in her 50s, frequently exclaimed 'Oh, not him! He's *boring*' and covered her ears with her hands. However, she was usually smiling while she did this. Similarly, Maggie, who was a particularly strong character within the group, often asked me what music I had brought along that week and said that if I played any pop songs she wasn't coming. Despite this, I would often see her sat at the back with Jean from where they would loudly appraise the music that was being played. It is likely that Maggie's attendance may have been motivated by a desire to socialise with others. However, it is also possible that attending these sessions gave her an opportunity to assert her identity by distinguishing herself from the 'popular' tastes of the group.

Berger's study on taste and divergence points to the possibilities of music in supporting the social life of a care home by creating both opportunities for inclusion and opportunities for residents to differentiate from each other. Finding strategies for responding creatively and democratically to these differences can be challenge for artists, particularly when working in group contexts. As this chapter has illustrated, differences in taste can also highlight social and cultural differences and lead to exclusion in an arts project. However, considering taste in terms of its social potential might open up new ways of thinking about how arts practices interact with the social life of the care home. Additionally, engaging with the diverse tastes of residents can create new aesthetic opportunities for arts practices in care homes.

Though many of the participants in the old film and music club were in their 80s and 90s, there were also several younger residents who took part who were in their mid to late 60s. Many of these residents were men who had moved to the care home due to a physical injury or illness which prevented them from living independently, such as a stroke or an amputation, or from substance-related mental health problems. These residents had grown up in the 1960s and 70s, and consequently their tastes were very different to that of the older residents. At the end of one of the music sessions I was approached by a heavily tattooed man who had been watching the workshop from outside the door. He asked me if I had any Santana or Jimi Hendrix and told me that he had played guitar himself before he had a stroke. His request for Jimi Hendrix surprised me. Not only did it emphasise the diversity of tastes within a care home, it drew attention to the fact that the tastes of care home residents are evolving with each generation.

Until recently, many of the arts practices that have taken place in care homes have been designed with the pre-war generation in mind. This is apparent in the popularity of reminiscence projects in the recent years which are themed around the war, tea dances and seaside holidays in Britain. For example, Age Exchange Theatre Trust's *Paddling to the Palais* (2013) which drew on the experiences of participants holidaying in British seaside towns in the 1930s and 1940s. While these experiences can be very meaningful for residents born in the 1920s and 30s, they will mean less to those who were born after the end of war. This point is taken up by Nicky Taylor, in her guide to dementia-friendly performances, where she observes 'Around 40,000 people in the UK are diagnosed with dementia before the age of 65, therefore a show which focuses on, for example, wartime memories will only be relevant for some of the audience' (Taylor 2016, p. 14). The changing tastes of the ageing population have aesthetic implications for arts practices in care homes, as it requires artists to engage with the cultural and social reference points that are meaningful to different generations.

The request for rock music by the younger resident at Mildmay reflected the importance of this genre for people who were young adults in the 1960s. This something which has also been picked up by the gerontologist Stephen Katz who suggests that rock music continues to be significant to the boomer generation, and particularly men, as they approach old age. '[Rock] Music has become the boomer generation's way of representing itself to itself as a collective, as it has moved through families, jobs, places, illnesses, and losses…. the generational pressure to keep classic rock timeless is connected to its ubiquity as an audionarrative that reiterates memories, relationships, and belongings as life-long experiences' (Katz 2014,

p. 1). The resident's love of Jimi Hendrix encouraged me to think about the social and aesthetic qualities of rock music and how it might be used to create new social experiences in a care community. In addition to understanding the changing needs of care home residents, rock music may offer artists an alternative means of representing the experiences of a new generation of older people.

This chapter explored how an arts project intersects with the politics of space in a care home, and how participation in an arts project can reveal a residents' position within a care home community. By examining some of the ways in which residents express personal tastes within a music and film project, it suggested that taste can be both a social resource which affords social capital and a source of tension, which highlights cultural and socio-economic differences. The practice examined in this chapter also challenged some common assumptions about taste in later life; the idea that older people will always be nostalgic the music from their youth, and the assumption that people from the same generation will like the same sort of music. Understanding how tastes can develop and change in later life is important when planning arts projects in care homes. As well as developing projects around personal tastes, artists have an opportunity to curate new experiences for residents, introducing them to art forms that they may not have encountered before and enabling them to cultivate new skills.

The previous two chapters looked at some of the ways in which artists can develop their practice around the sensory and social qualities of a care home. In the last of the practice-based chapters, I will look a little more closely at the creative contributions of people living with dementia and how performance practitioners might use them as a starting point for collaboration.

Note

1. One such project is 'Men in Sheds', a project which uses woodwork and other activities to support older men (www.ageuk.org.uk).

References

Bennett, A. (2013). *Music, Style and Ageing: Growing Old Disgracefully?* Philadelphia: Temple University Press.

Bennett, A., & Taylor, J. (2012). Popular Music and the Aesthetics of Ageing. *Popular Music, 31*(2), 231–243.

Berger, J., Heath, C., & Ho, B. (2007). *Divergence in Cultural Practices: Tastes as Signals of Identity*. Unpublished dissertation, Stamford University.

Bottero, W. (2009). Relationality and Social Interaction. *British Journal of Sociology, 60*(2), 399–420.

Bourdieu, P. (1984). *Distinction*. Oxon: Routledge.

Bourdieu, P. (1986). The Forms of Capital. In J. Richardson (Ed.), *Handbook of Theory and Research for the Sociology of Education* (pp. 241–258). New York: Greenwood.

Cornell, M. (2012). Talking about Old Records: Generational Musical Identity among Older People. *Popular Music, 31*(2), 261–278.

Daly, M, and Rake, K. (2003). *Gender and the Welfare State: Care, Work and Welfare in Europe and the USA*. Cambridge: Polity Press.

DiMaggio, P. (1987). Classifications in Art. *American Sociological Review. 52*(2), 440–450.

Forman, M. (2012). 'How We Feel the Music': Popular Music by Elders and for Elders'. *Popular Music, 31*(2), 245–260.

Harrison, J., & Ryan, J. (2010). Musical Taste and Ageing. *Ageing & Society, 30*, 649–669.

Hebdige, D. (1979). *Subculture: the Meaning of Style*. London: Routledge.

Katz, S. (2014). Music, Performance and Generation: The Making of Boomer Rock and Roll Biographies. In C. Harrington, D. Bielby, & A. Bardo (Eds.), *Aging, Media, Culture* (pp. 93–106). New York: Lexington Press.

Kjellman-Chapin, M. (2013). *Kitsch: History, Theory, Practice*. Durham, NC: Duke University Press.

Kontos, P. (2005). Embodied Selfhood in Alzheimer's Disease: Rethinking Person-Centred Care. *Dementia, 4*(4), 553–570.

Miller, D. (2009). *The Comfort of Things*. London: Polity Press.

Nicholson, H. (2011). Making Home Work: Theatre Making with Older Adults in Residential Care. *NJ: Drama Australia Journal, 35*(1), 47–62.

Perry, G. (2012). *In the Best Possible Taste with Grayson Perry*. Documentary Series, Channel 4, 2012. Retrieved October 8, 2017, from http://www.channel4.com/programmes/in-the-best-possible-taste-grayson-perry/

Segal, L. (2014). *Out of Time: The Perils and Pleasures of Ageing*. London: Verso.

Skeggs, B. (2006). *Class, Self, Culture*. London: Routledge.

Smith, K. (2000). Mere Nostalgia: Notes on a Progressive Paratheory. *Rhetoric and Public Affairs, 3*(4), 505–527.

Taylor, N. (2016). *West Yorkshire Playhouse's Guide to Dementia Friendly Performances*. Leeds: West Yorkshire Playhouse.

Twigg, J., & Buse, C. (2013). Dress, Dementia and the Embodiment of Identity. *Dementia, 12*(3), 326–336.

CHAPTER 7

Taking Care: A Methodology for Collaboration

This chapter is about collaboration and the ways in which practices of performance and care can overlap in a care home. It departs from my own practice, offering an analysis of STORYBOX, an improvisational storytelling programme for older people, with a particular focus on those living with dementia. STORYBOX is run by Small Things Creative Projects, who are based in Manchester, but work in care homes across the UK. My analysis of their work is centred on some of the ways in which creativity occurs as part of daily life in a care home, and how the artists engage with these small, everyday acts of creativity. Rather than thinking of arts practices in care homes in terms of their transformative potential, this chapter considers collaboration as two types of creative practice meeting in the middle.

In drawing out the particular qualities that are required of artists for this type of collaboration to occur, I have returned to some of Martin Welton's work on 'feeling theatre', specifically his analysis of *Common Dance*. *Common Dance* was a community dance production created by the choreographer Rosemary Lee in 2009. It explored, among other things, how practices and qualities of care can manifest within a performance process. By weaving an analysis of STORYBOX with *Common Dance*, I hope to form the beginnings of a methodology for collaboration in care homes which is based on reciprocity and attention. I start with some reflections on a STORYBOX workshop in order to illustrate how this type of collaboration can work in practice.

N. Hatton, *Performance and Dementia*,
https://doi.org/10.1007/978-3-030-51077-0_7

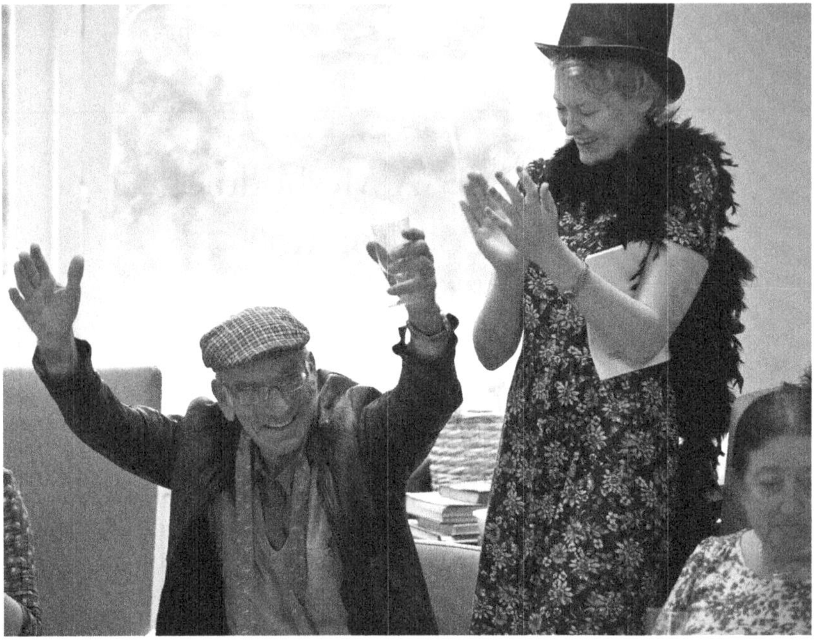

Fig. 7.1 STORYBOX workshop featuring Sara Cocker and STORYBOX participants. (Photograph by Roshana Rubin Mayhew for Small Things Creative Projects)

It is a typically drizzly morning in South Manchester and I am spending the day with artists Lowri Evans and Sara Cocker. We have arrived at Meadow View: a large, private care facility near the border of the Peak District. The site is a sprawling complex of old buildings, each of which are named, unironically, after British Royal residences (Balmoral, Sandringham, Craigowan, Windsor). This morning's workshop is taking place at Balmoral—a building which mainly accommodates residents with dementia.

In the previous session the residents shared memories about going to Belle Vue—a fairground and zoo that was a popular attraction in Manchester in the 1940s and 50s. Their recollections have inspired the theme for today's workshop and we have arrived in a car that is crammed full to the roof with fairground paraphernalia including, cock-a-hoop rings, coconuts, sparkly hats, balloons, and 'goldfish' prizes (carrot sticks in bags of water). Today's workshop is taking place on Remembrance Day and the staff aren't sure how many residents will want to take part. We enter a long, narrow conservatory surrounded by a well-kept lawn. At one end there is a lounge area with three or four armchairs arranged around a television. At the other end residents sit in chairs around the edge of the space, a little distance away from each other. I wonder how Lowri and Sara will address the group as a whole as everyone is so spread out. There are no care staff to be seen and it would be difficult to move the residents without help as most of them are seated in heavy-backed armchairs. A breakfast television programme blares into the room and some residents are watching it attentively. One woman is reading a TV magazine. She looks up and nods at us when we enter the room, then goes back to her magazine. A couple of residents are sleeping. I make eye contact with a man at the far end of the room who grins at me and gives me a little wave.

Lowri and Sara start to unpack, placing props and pieces of costume around the room and greeting people warmly as they go. Some of the residents watch them with faint interest and comment on the props. Others ignore them and focus on the TV. I am half expecting a member of staff to arrive and formally introduce us but no one comes. When everything is unpacked and they have greeted every resident individually, Lowri suggests turning the TV off. The woman with the magazine looks up and responds with a firm 'no thank you'. Another resident shouts out from the other side of the room: 'Where has that bitch gone? She's gone and left me here'. As Sara crosses the room to speak to her Lowri turns to me and whispers, 'I think today might be difficult. I think we're going to have to go with it'. Unsure of how to proceed, we sit down rather awkwardly and watch TV with the residents.

A little before 11 am, a member of care staff arrives and fiddles with a wreath of paper poppies, trying to hang it up in the window. After a while she gives up and props it against the wall. She walks over to the TV and switches the channel to the BBC coverage of Remembrance Day. On seeing her, the woman who shouted begins to call out again. The carer pats her hand and says a couple of reassuring words before leaving the room. The woman focuses her attention on Sara and tells her that they have taken her away from her family. Sara perches on the arm of her chair and takes her hand. At 11 am the TV prompts us all into a two-minute silence. All eyes are glued to the screen and the room is suddenly very still. Towards the end of the silence the television camera accidentally catches some MPs in suits talking through it. A couple of the residents snigger and the mood lifts a little. When it has finished, Lowri takes the opportunity to turn the volume down and asks if anyone would like some music. After what feels like a very long pause, the man who waved at me gestures towards her blue cowboy boots and says 'these boots were made for walking'. Lowri says she has 'just the song' and Sara searches for it on her iPod. As Nancy Sinatra's voice drifts into the space, some of the residents begin to nod their heads to the beat. The woman with the TV magazine looks up with recognition. Lowri leads them into a warm-up exercise, inviting them to do a series of stretches, stomps and hand gestures in time to the music. As she moves, Sara goes around each resident individually, offering them her hands and helping them to raise their arms higher in the air. The song ends and another one starts. This time Lowri goes around the room inviting each resident to pick a movement for the rest of the group to copy. The activity coordinator decides that this is a good time to water all of the plants in the conservatory and zig-zags across the space with a jug, spilling water and talking loudly as she goes.

Finding the Sense of a Beginning

In *The Philosophy of Improvisation*, Gary Peters addresses the difficulty that improvisers can face in finding 'the sense of a beginning' (Peters 2009, p. 1). This difficulty, he suggests, stems from the fact that a decisive beginning may only be established after a 'multitude of false starts, erasures and abortive attempts to get things going' (ibid.). Finding the sense of a beginning involves understanding how it is 'entangled' with these previous attempts to get started, as well as finding a way of engaging with the moment. Peters' suggestion may be applicable to most instances of improvising or devising performance but is particularly relevant to the process of getting started in a care home. Knowing how and when to start a workshop can involve a lot of uncertainty as artists must be responsive to what is happening in the space at that particular time. In this instance, the fact that the workshop was taking place on Remembrance Day meant that it started with the artists sitting down and watching TV with the residents. So at what point did the creative 'work' begin? When the TV got turned down? When the resident commented on Lowri's boots? When we watched Remembrance Day coverage together? Or earlier still, before we entered the room? In addition to the planning and preparation that took place days or even weeks before the workshop began, the difficulty of pinpointing the start of the creative work seemed in part due to the fact that there were different types of creative activity taking place in the room. On first appearance, it may seem that a care home is inherently lacking in creative activity. The image of older people sitting in armchairs facing the television is a dominant stereotype, associated with a lack of occupation or the ability of residents to engage in more 'meaningful' activities. The journalist Valentine Low writing in *The Times* evokes the apparent passivity that is often associated with this stereotype. 'The image that springs to mind is of a large communal room with chairs arranged around the perimeter, television blaring in a corner while the residents sit with blank, lifeless expressions' (Low 2013). However, if I reflect on what the residents were doing when we arrived at Meadow View, it seemed that there was a lot of creative activity taking place. This was apparent in the way that they attended to their individual routines within the communal environment of the lounge. For the woman with the TV magazine, reading was a strategy which enabled her to participate selectively in group activities. I noticed that she chose to stay in the lounge for the duration of STORYBOX workshop and participated in some of the exercises. However, the magazine gave her an excuse to sit out the activities that she did not want to do and participate on her own terms.

Opening up to the creativity of these personal routines involves, I suggest, embracing the fuzziness that exists around 'getting started' and recognising that the creative practice of artists is entangled with the creative practice of everyday life in a care home. In approaching this task, I am mindful that this type of collaboration will never be evenly balanced. Residents often have little choice about whether to attend a workshop, particularly when it is taking place in a communal space. However, by taking the creative practices of everyday life as a starting point, artists may challenge a perception of participatory arts where residents need to be 'rescued' from the monotony of the care home and move towards a relational approach, which acknowledges the creativity that is inherent in their everyday lives.

Creativity in Everyday Life

> The forward movement of keeping going ... can involve a good measure of creative improvisation, not unlike that required of pedestrians on a busy street ... one's own movement is attuned on the one hand to that of companions who one wishes to keep abreast or in file, and on the other, to strangers coming from different directions with whom one does not wish to collude. (Hallam and Ingold 2008, p. 7)

In *Creativity and Cultural Improvisation* the anthropologists Elizabeth Hallam and Tim Ingold argue that improvisation is part of everyday life, an integral aspect of how people negotiate social situations in a world which is 'continually in the making' (ibid.: 2). People must improvise due to the fact that 'there is no script for social and cultural life', which means they must 'work it out as they go along' (ibid.: 1). They go on to outline the relational nature of cultural improvisation, suggesting that it involves 'mutually constitutive relationships' through which humans 'continually participate in each other's coming-into-being (ibid.). Rather than being an artistic skill which is learnt through years of training, cultural improvisation is woven into the mundane practices of everyday life and traced through everyday encounters between people.

The concept of cultural improvisation is instructive in understanding how residents negotiate or 'attune' to different social situations in a care home. This task can be especially challenging for residents as they are frequently required to acclimatise to 'strangers coming from different directions'. In a care home, these strangers might include a flow of care staff, residents, health workers, family members, artists and activity workers that frequent the home on a regular basis. For people with dementia, the task of 'keeping going' can be especially difficult, as the social encounter they find themselves in may be unfamiliar. As a regular visitor to a care home, I have noticed that residents with dementia will often adopt the type of conversational patterns that are associated with receiving visitors in the home as a strategy for approaching these encounters. I have often had residents initiate a conversation with me by commenting on the weather or asking if I have had far to travel this morning. One resident at Meadow View said 'it's nice to see you again', even though it was the first time that we had met. Her awareness that I was a visitor whom she might have met before and forgotten, and her ability to improvise around this, indicated a particular type of creativity akin to Hallam and Ingold's concept of improvisation. Another example of this type of improvisation was the way that some of the residents told stories from their long-term past as a means of stimulating a conversation. In the STORYBOX workshop, a man who I was sat next to asked me if I liked horses. When I said yes, he proceeded to tell me that he had trained horses throughout his life, starting when he was 15 years old. It struck me that his question was a way in to a conversation about a topic that he knew he could be conversant about, one that didn't rely on his short-term memory. The resourcefulness with which people with dementia improvise in social situations is one example of everyday creativity in a care home. This type of creativity is also visible within the more mundane practices of everyday life.

Television and Homemaking

The television is widely considered, and with reasonable justification, to be a negative aspect of care home life. Low's description of residents sitting in rows facing the television is certainly consistent with my first experience of a care home, and the challenges that I encountered communicating over the noise. There have also been several studies which consider the negative impact that television can have on those living with dementia. These include Kate de Medeiros et al. (2009), who consider the behavioural effects of television and J.S. Shin et al. (2013), who assess the impact that excessive television-watching may have on those living with fronto-temporal dementia. However, my experience of watching television with the residents at Meadow View prompted me to think about it differently. As my time at Mildmay indicated, television can offer residents an element of choice in an environment where there is little choice available. When I switched off the TV in order to play film footage during the music sessions, resident Rose would frequently protest. This was not the passive, sedentary behaviour that is often associated with watching television in care homes. Similarly, the residents at Meadow View were not watching the Remembrance Day coverage passively. They were actively focused on the ceremony. For many of them, the coverage may have stimulated a connection to a significant event in their pasts as well as connections to friends, family members, and places outside of the care home. For those with dementia, making sense of this coverage may have involved connecting up different places, times and events both recent and in the distant past. The routine act of watching television in a care home may be an important way that people with dementia contextualise their world in an environment that is unfamiliar. To my knowledge there has been no research which explores the potential of television in supporting people with dementia to make connections with other places, people or events in their lives. My observations of the residents watching Remembrance Day coverage suggests that this is worthy of further investigation.

Another interpretation is that watching television is an important aspect of home-making in a care home, as it is a continuation of a domestic routine that residents may have enjoyed before they moved there. Kerstin Mackley and Sarah Pink support this idea in their ethnographical study of night-time domestic routines in the UK. In their article *Moving, Making and Atmosphere*, they describe how 'everyday atmospheres of home are made, maintained and improvised through habitual routines of movement' (Mackley and Pink 2014, p. 1). Describing how their participants subconsciously turned lights on and off during their night-time routines, they suggest that certain domestic routines are carried out in order to create a 'sensory aesthetic of home' (ibid.: 2). Rather than seeing these routines as mundane or unremarkable, they argue that they represent 'skilled ways of knowing and improvisatory tendencies in the everyday tasks of home' (ibid.: 6).

Although the domestic activity taking place in their study is different, their analysis is applicable to television-watching in a care home, which may be conceived as a creative act when thought of as an improvised form of home-making. In the same way that their participants subconsciously altered the lighting within their home environment, it could be argued that the practice of watching television, or being present when the television is on, is a way that care home residents re-create a sensory aesthetic of home. In addition to continuing with a domestic routine, the television may offer a familiar soundscape for residents that is associated with home. For Amir at Mildmay, the routine of watching *Columbo* in the lounge at the same time everyday certainly seemed to be associated with relaxation, as he would do so at a time when he knew he would be undisturbed by other residents. The punctuality of this routine, combined with the sensory experience of watching and listening to his favourite programme may have been a strategy that enabled him to re-create a sense of home in a communal area. Furthermore, it may have helped to create a sense of purpose in his day.

Sleeping and Social Retreat

Sleeping is an activity which takes place frequently in communal care spaces as well as in bedrooms. It is an activity that can occur on and off throughout the day, often in the presence of other people and at the same time as other activities. Sleep is a particularly important part of the daily routine of residents who are living with dementia. The Alzheimer's Society suggest that people who are living with the late stages of dementia typically spend 40 per cent of their time in bed at night awake and a significant part of their daytime sleeping (alz.org). The prevalence of sleeping in communal spaces raises questions about its significance as a part of everyday life in a care home. Rather than dismissing it as a sedentary activity, or an activity to pass the time, exploring how residents negotiate sleep within different social and spatial contexts may reveal its potential as a creative act.

The human geographers Peter Kraftl and John Horton believe there is a need to pay attention to sleep as a critical aspect of human geography. They describe sleep as a 'fundamentally spatial and spatially-produced phenomenon' (Kraftl and Horton 2008, p. 510), and consider it as an '(in)active agent in the construction of multifarious spaces and spatialities' (ibid.: 520). Their attention to space is pertinent to how sleep may be employed by residents to negotiate personal space within a care home. Kraftl and Horton argue that sleep plays a fundamental role in 'producing and delimiting the everyday time-space rhythms and rituals of most human beings (ibid.: 512), suggesting that sleep may be a way of structuring the day and creating personal boundaries within communal spaces. Considered in this way, sleep may be understood as a strategy which is used by residents to avoid certain social situations or activities. An example that springs to mind is a carol concert that I attended at a care home shortly before Christmas. All residents were encouraged to attend the concert and although some residents seemed to enjoy it, many of them dozed through it. I couldn't help wonder if their sleeping was, in part, a form of protest at being encouraged to attend the concert. My experience was echoed by Murray Forman who, in researching musical performances in care homes, observed that 'residents at each facility were wheeled into the performance rooms … whether they cared for the music or not' (Forman 2012, p. 251). He noticed that the residents who were 'prone to sleep' through the musical performances were spoken about 'slightly disparagingly' by staff, while those who 'tapped their fingers or toes to the rhythm, sang along or even danced' were 'subtly praised' (ibid.: 252). Forman's observations on sleeping during scheduled activities draw attention to the possibilities of sleep as a form of resistance to the regulatory practices of care settings.

In considering the creative potential of sleep in care homes, I have been inspired by some anthropological research on daytime napping in Japanese culture. In a study of Japanese politicians who sleep through parliament, the anthropologist Bridgette Steger uses the term 'inemuri', a word which literally translates as 'to be asleep while present' (Steger 2003, p. 181) to describe how politicians will frequently sleep on the job. Rather than being seen as form of laziness, *inemuri* is considered to be an indication of hard work as employees are working too hard to get enough sleep at home.

Inemuri is considered to be a legitimate form of 'social retreat' within Japanese culture which enables a person to rest while continuing to be socially present (sleepers will typically remain in an upright position in order to show that they are still socially engaged in some way).

I have been in several workshops in care homes where participants have fallen asleep for some or for all of it. In many circumstances this would be seen a failure on behalf of the artist to engage their participants. However, following Steger, sleep may also be understood as a strategic tool in a care home which enables residents to engage selectively with the activities of the care home. Though her study offers a very culturally specific way of thinking about sleep as a creative activity, the concept of *inemuri* is instructive here as it suggests that residents can still be asleep and 'socially present' in a workshop, even if they are not participating in the activities.

Applying creative readings to the everyday routines of care home residents broadens our understanding of what they can contribute to the artistic process. By looking beyond the daytime routines of residents as a way of passing the time, artists may begin to understand the creative ways in which residents negotiate everyday life in a care home. However, the task of identifying and engaging with these everyday activities can be challenging for artists. How do artists engage creatively with these activities without imposing their own creative practice? In the next part of the chapter I attempt to identify the processes involved in engaging with the everyday creativity of care homes, and offer a methodology for collaboration.

The Creativity of Care

My methodology starts with the idea of care as a creative practice. It suggests that the concept of care, when looked at under the lens of performance studies, may help artists to engage with the everyday creativity of a care home. The phrase 'taking care' has several connotations: of looking after a person, of being cautious, of keeping oneself safe, and of approaching a task or activity in an attentive way. Martin Welton has used this latter definition of care to consider the way in which performers attend to different tasks and activities in rehearsal and performance. In an article that precedes *Feeling Theatre*, he forges a direct connection between care and attention in the work of the choreographer Rosemary Lee. Drawing on Lee's production *Common Dance*, he suggests that that the care with which a performer engages with a particular task, or with another performer, may be interpreted as a 'mode of attention' (Welton 2010, p. 48).

Welton's interpretation of care as a mode of attention in performance is central to my approach. It suggests that the process of engaging with everyday spaces requires a particular type of attention to what is happening in the room. By conceptualising care as an attentive act, rather than a generic quality that artists need when working in care homes, I hope to demonstrate how artists attend creatively to the practices of everyday life in a care home. Furthermore, the concept of care as a mode of attention raises questions as to how residents and artists attend to each other in different ways.

Common Dance was a large-scale, intergenerational production which featured as part of the Dance Umbrella International Festival in 2009. The piece features an ensemble of mostly non-professional dancers of different ages, and a children's choir, in a performance that Welton described as 'a diverse group of people paying attention to each other' (ibid.: 47). The production was subsequently the subject of a symposium, *On Taking Care*, where performance scholars and practitioners interviewed Lee about the themes and processes attached to the piece. What interests me about *Common Dance*, and Lee's reflections on it, are the connections that she makes between care and artistic creation. For Lee, the concept of 'taking care' described the relationship between company members as well as the motifs of the performance. Care was a recurring image in the production and the repeated sequences of performers lifting, guiding and gently supporting each other gave the production a caring aesthetic. Lee explains that these tactile explorations were also an integral aspect of how the ensemble learned to work together as a company. In film footage of the first rehearsal, the performers are encouraged to get to know each other through a series of gentle physical encounters, such as leading each other by the hand to explore different parts of the room. She explains: 'the relationship between caring for someone feels quite similar to me in terms of when you're caring to bring forth a piece.... I was really interested in that place, that moment ... the whole thing of being present' (Lee 2012).

This occupation with care as both a process and an image in *Common Dance* feels like an appropriate place to start when considering how artists and participants collaborate in care homes. How might practices of care in large-scale ensemble performances inform creative collaborations of a more intimate scale in care homes? If I reflect on the STORYBOX workshop, I can recall different types of care-taking from the way that Sara comforted the resident who was distressed by holding her hand, to the way in which the residents attended to the creative tasks of the workshop.

Whether this care was about meeting an emotional need or the way that someone approached a particular activity, the quality of attention was the same. This is an observation which is shared by both Lee and Welton in their analysis of *Common Dance*.

At the beginning of *Common Dance*, the performers are curled up on the floor of the space with their eyes closed. The audience walk through and around the motionless bodies to take their seats. They must take care with their steps, watching out for fingers, hair and other body parts that they might tread or trip up on. After they have taken their seats, some of the younger performers begin to wake up, stretching and slowly uncurling. They crawl purposefully and silently to the older members of the company and gently place their heads on their bodies, listening carefully, perhaps for a heartbeat or a breath. Slowly, they begin to coax them out of their sleep, using their heads and noses to nuzzle their limbs into wakefulness. The task, which takes a good few minutes, is undertaken with great care and attention. The image of heads cocked closely on the body recurs throughout the performance, and creates the feeling that the performers are listening attentively to each other's bodies.

Attention is the focus of Welton's analysis of *Common Dance* and one which he connects directly to the practice of 'taking care'. For him, taking care was visible in the ways that the performers attended to each other's bodies in this opening sequence but also in the relationship that they had to the work itself. He describes a particular moment in the performance where 'in laying hands on one another, moving and being moved by one another lifting each other with great care, paying attention was both the mode and matter of their performance' (Welton 2010, p. 47). Considering the particular connection between care and attention, he describes it as a process of listening:

> Listening conceived as mode of touch might offer a means of describing the experience of performance in terms of 'paying attention'—a mode of attention in which one is reciprocally giving as well as receiving… The show made space for listening as a treatment in the sense of both a handling of and a quality of care. (Ibid.)

I have suggested that working creatively with care homes requires a particular type of engagement, a sort of attunement to what is taking place in the space at that particular time. Welton's concept of listening points to some of the different ways that artists may tune in to a care space. One of the ways that this might happen is by them joining in with the activities of the space, as Lowri and Sara did when they watched the Remembrance Day ceremony together. Another example is the way that artists attend to the contributions of the residents. When the resident commented on Lowri's boots, she attended to his suggestion by playing the song 'These boots are made for walking'. This process of 'saying yes' to whatever is offered is a fundamental aspect of the STORYBOX approach, and is a good example of how artist pay creative attention to what the residents offer. However, Welton's concept of listening as a mode of attention, and listening to bodies in particular, is significant to how artists pay attention somatically in a care home. This has particular resonance for working with residents who are non-verbal and may contribute in different ways. In this context, paying attention might mean paying attention to a particular movement or sound that a resident does habitually and incorporating it into the work.

The improvisational storytelling programme, *Timeslips*, created by Anne Basting, offers a good example of this sort of practice. Basting created *Timeslips* after working with people at the later stages of dementia. She was interested in developing a form of storytelling which captured 'the complexity of their worlds and our relationship to them … complete with missing words, repeated sounds and hazy memories' (Basting 2001, p. 79). Rather than encouraging participants to recall stories from the past, the purpose was to create new stories from imagination through a process of collaborative storytelling. In a *Timeslips* workshop every verbal contribution that is offered is incorporated into the story. Basting explains that, 'all answers were folded into the story. One storyteller, whose language was limited to sounds, offered "Babababababa." It became part of nearly every story we told' (ibid.: 6). Her example demonstrated that the process of 'paying attention' or 'listening' to the contributions of people with dementia involves accepting them in the form they are expressed. I would like to expand this idea by considering the different types of creative contributions that people with dementia make, and how artists attend to them creatively. For people with dementia who are non-verbal, creative contributions may be physical, such a facial expression, a gesture, or a form of physical contact with the facilitator or another participant. As such, the process of engagement needs to be understood not just through listening but also through notions of touch. In understanding what the rehearsal space offered to the performer, Welton described the affordances that an actress receives from the sensation of her foot on the stage as a 'condition of feeling' (Welton 2010, p. 106). I propose that this condition of feeling also goes some way to understanding the non-verbal contributions that are made by people with dementia, and the tactile exchanges that take place during these moments.

Tactile Engagements

Earlier in this book I discussed the type of exchanges that might take place as part of a relational framework for dementia care. The concept of 'feeling theatre' was introduced in order to understand the sensory and emotional qualities that both parties should experience within a caregiving relationship. The emphasis on the feeling qualities of relational care are instructive in considering how artist and participants engage with each other through sensory and tactile experiences.

The physical interactions that took place between the performers of *Common Dance* demonstrated how they alternately engaged and found themselves engaged through touch. This process was visible in the opening sequence of the performance when the younger members of the company engaged the older members by nuzzling them with their heads. Lee explains that this 'somatic approach' was integral to the devising process, as sequences of dance were developed from tasks which connected the performers through hand-to-body contact.

Lee's discussion of the 'somatic approach' is similar to what Welton describes as 'motility' in *Feeling Theatre*. Welton uses the word motility to describe 'the condition and feeling of being in motion' (ibid.: 107) as opposed to mobility, the ability to be able to move. Rather than focusing on the range or the type of movement that a performer is doing, Lee describes the somatic approach as 'the experience of movement … how they feel it with whatever senses they have' (Lee 2012). This type of feeling engagement, whether it is between performers or with a space itself, is useful in considering the reciprocity of the creative relationship in a care home. Specifically, how people with dementia might engage artists creatively through touch.

A few years ago I participated in a performance called *Paddling to the Palais* which was run by Age Exchange Theatre Trust. The project was led by composer Natasha Lohan and dancer Stella Howard, and involved older people from the local area, some who were living with dementia, and their family carers. The weekly sessions combined movement, sound and reminiscence with the aim of devising a group piece of work that would be performed in the final week. After attending for a few weeks I noticed that Pat, a woman with dementia, would always offer to warm up the hands of the person next to her by rubbing them between her own. When the artists realised this they decided to incorporate the gesture into the physical warm up each week so that *everyone* got their hands rubbed. Rubbing hands was Pat's way of making visitors feel welcome as they entered the space, engaging them through touch and through the temperature of her hands. In turn, the artists' decision to replicate her gesture in the group warm up was a way of acknowledging Pat's contribution in a creative way.

Lee talks about this reciprocity of tactile encounters in her own work. Asked about the tactile relationship she has with the performers she works with, she explains that touch is a way of engaging them both: '[I think it's] something about wanting to make people feel at home and reassured ... a hand on a knee or a shoulder ... [but it also] helps me feel connected, not separate' (ibid.). Her belief that she needs to feel physically connected to her participants in order to be engaged is important to my methodology as it reiterates the need for artists to experience a feeling of care in order to do the work. Care of the artist is something which I will discuss in more detail in the following section in relation to emotional labour. However, it is worth mentioning at this point that a creative collaboration in a care home involves understanding the different ways in which residents care for artists. These types of tactile encounter demonstrate the vital role that residents play in helping artists to experience a feeling of care, as well as the unique contributions that people with dementia make to a creative partnership.

Creating a methodology that is based on reciprocity rather than transformation requires some re-examination of the concept of engagement in participatory theatre. Traditionally, the word 'engagement' has been associated with community participation. In working towards an early definition of applied theatre, for example, Philip Taylor wrote that 'applied theatre engages participants in an important conversation about issues directly experienced in their community' (Taylor 2003, p. xxix). Embedded within the early history of Theatre in Education in the UK is idea of theatre as a method of engagement in schools and the association of engagement with learning has fed into the development of several 'learning and engagement departments' in theatres in the UK.[1] In *Engaging Performance*, Jan Cohen-Cruz explores the connotations and evolution of the term. Contesting the idea of engagement as a unidirectional process, she foregrounds the '*relationships* at the heart of making art with such aspirations and dependence on a genuine exchange between artist and community'. (Cohen-Cruz 2010, p. 7, her emphasis). When examined closely, the term 'engagement' can be understood as relational in character in that it can refer to both the act of engaging someone and the act of being engaged. The word also connotes varying degrees of involvement, from getting someone's attention to securing their active involvement in a task or activity. The relationship between an audience member's engagement and the engagement of the performer in the task they are doing is a process that performance writer Matilda Leyser describes as 'becoming engaged in their doing' (Leyser 2012). Her interpretation is helpful in considering the processes in which artists identify and work with the everyday creativity of care home residents. In addition to their attempts to engage residents in the creative activities they have prepared, they must also be attuned to the creative activity that is already present in the room.

The geographers Ben Anderson Paul Harrison describe attunement as a process of 'inhabiting'. 'We come to know and enact a world from inhabiting it, from becoming attuned to its differences and juxtapositions, from a training of our senses, dispositions and expectations and from being able to initiate, imitate and elaborate skilled lines of action. (Anderson and Harrison 2010, p. 9). Their definition is instructive in understanding the sensory intuition and embodied attention that is necessary for artists to engage with the creative activity of a care home. In STORYBOX, the start of the workshop was affected by Remembrance Day and the fact that the residents were watching the ceremony on television. Instead of attempting to introduce the activities they had prepared around this, Lowri and Sara understood the importance of watching the ceremony together on the TV. By tuning in to the coverage, they were also tuning in to the everyday activities of the space. The moment suggested that paying attention in a creative sense also involves a process of attuning to the spatial and temporal rhythms of a care community.

Paying Attention

Lee and Welton's analysis of *Common Dance* indicates that care can be a mode of attention, both between performers and in the relationship they have to the performance itself. An important consideration for performance in care homes is how participants pay attention in different ways. At Meadow View some of the participants were deaf, some had dementia and others had physical impairments which affected how they attended to the workshop activities. In order to establish the feasibility of this approach in a care home, it is necessary to consider how residents tune in to the workshop in different ways. Paying attention to these individual needs may not always be as straightforward as acknowledging what someone has said. It might involve physical modes of attention, such as hand-to-body contact or paying attention to sound and breath, rather than to words. Exploring how artists and residents pay attention to each other in different ways may offer a more nuanced understanding of creative collaboration in a dementia care context.

The task of tuning into individual modes of attention while still attending to the group as a whole can be challenging as artists must find a way of balancing the individual needs of the participants with the needs of the group. The way that the STORYBOX workshop was co-facilitated by Lowri and Sara offered some insight into how this might be approached. Throughout the workshop, a relay-type relationship was used in which they swapped between group and one-to-one work. When Lowri led the group in a physical warm-up, Sara worked individually with participants, moving around the circle and adapting the exercises where necessary to suit their needs. Sometimes this meant doing something quite different to what the rest of the circle were doing. For example, one man associated the music that was playing with his ballroom dancing days and preferred to talk to Sara about this rather than copying the movements. In the next exercise they would swap over so that Sara led the group and Lowri worked one-on-one. This technique enabled them to attend to the individual needs of the participants while still maintaining a forward momentum to the session. It also enabled them to get to know the residents and find out information that might inform a future activity. Through working on-one-one with the man who had gone ballroom dancing, Sara was able to find out about the sort of music he liked to dance to and was able to source some of the pieces for the following week.

Sometimes, the way in which they attended to an individual need was demonstrated by a physical type of attention. When the resident was visibly distressed and confused at the beginning of the workshop, Sara responded by sitting very close beside her and holding her hand. After a few minutes, this woman did not want to let go of her hand so Sara led exercises while perched on the arm of her chair for the rest of the session. Her attention to this resident's needs was represented through this continuous physical contact—a gesture which felt similar to what Welton refers to as 'marrying listening with touch' (Welton 2010, p. 50). In addition to 'listening' to her anxiety by holding her hand, Sara's physical connection to her while she was facilitating was of a way of continuing to include her in the creative process. This moment affirmed Lee's suggestion that the process of care-taking in a 'looking after' sense is closely related to the care-taking that occurs as part of a creative process.

In considering engagement as a tactile experience between performers, I am interested in how people with dementia engage others in a workshop. Certain types of tactile engagement can draw attention to the embodied creativity of people with dementia, as well as supporting them as leaders of artistic activities. During the physical warm-up at Meadow View I found myself paired with a man who had dementia. As music piped out from a tinny speaker, we silently touched hands at the finger tips. At first our fingers moved tentatively from side to side using a very small range of movement. The man was sunk back in his wheelchair and though his fingertips were engaged with mine, the rest of his body, including his arms, were slackened and heavy against the chair. Unsure of his physical abilities and not wanting to cause any discomfort or injury, I was cautious not to coax his arms too high or too far out to the side. We carried on in this way for a while, moving our arms gently back and forward in a horizontal motion, until, after a while, we made eye contact and held each other's gaze. After this, we became more confident. Our palms slid together and started to move in slow circles. With each circle we went a little higher, stretching our arms further in the air. The sequence of movements prompted him to straighten his back which in turn moved his head and shoulders into an upright position. Our movements became faster and I realised that he was guiding me through the movements, applying gentle pressure to my palms and encouraging me to stretch my arms further.

When asked about the prevalence of hand-to-body contact in *Common Dance*, Lee talks about the 'intelligence of the hands' and 'how quickly you can affect change through the use of touch' (Lee 2012). She talks about the capacity of the hands to provoke movement or action in other areas of the body, claiming 'there is something in the doing they enable'. Her focus on the intelligence of the hands in a dance context resonated with my own experience of hand-to-hand contact with this resident. The tactile encounter between our fingertips opened up our awareness to the possibilities of movement in our arms, as well stimulating movement in other areas of our bodies, such as our spines, our shoulders and our heads. There was something about the way that we communicated through the hands and the fingertips which felt more attuned than the verbal communication we had attempted earlier in the session, which had felt slightly awkward. The experience demonstrated the type of creative engagements that people with dementia can instigate through physical contact as well as the potential of tactile engagements in supporting them as leaders of creative activities.

Combining individual and group facilitation is one strategy that artists may use to acknowledge the individual contributions of care home residents. However, there is a question as to how these contributions are taken forward or incorporated into the artistic process. The ability to take forward an individual contribution and incorporate it into the creative journey requires artists to be skilled improvisers, adapting and responding to whatever material they are given. Lowri and Sara told me that one of the most important aspects of the STORYBOX process is to 'say yes' to everything that is offered by the residents, in the same way that an improviser would say yes by accepting the previous line that is offered to them by another actor. People with dementia often improvise as part of their everyday lives, and the basic practice of 'saying yes' in dramatic improvisations is a strategy that can support their participation in an arts project without fear of failure. In the workshop at Meadow View, the process of 'saying yes' to the residents took different forms, from using an idea in a group exercise, to copying a particular gesture or sound, or joining in with a song that a resident was singing. 'Saying yes' often led to rich creative discoveries. When one resident said that he remembered riding the ghost train at Belle Vue, Lowri and Sara encouraged the group to create a soundscape that was made up of things you would find on a ghost train. The exercise demonstrated that 'saying yes' is not just about acknowledging the contribution of the resident in the way that it is given. It is finding a creative way in which to take it forward. This is not to say that every contribution must be developed into something much more substantial. Sometimes a resident reciting a song would end in a round of applause before the workshop moved on to something else. However, taking up these contributions was one way in which Lowri and Sara supported the residents to decide the content of the workshops. In the STORYBOX evaluation, they describe this process as 'levelling the playing field … so that the participants can shape the direction' (Harris 2013, p. 35).

In exploring how artists find imaginative ways of taking up the suggestions of the participants, it is important to consider the type of labour involved in this type of work. The process of saying yes to everything can be exhausting for the artist as it is a mode of attention which requires them to be continually responsive. As Sara reflected, you have to be 'constantly thinking on your feet, improvising, going with what the group give you' (Cocker 2014). Lowri and Sara run STORYBOX workshops in character but slip in and out as needed. For example, they might communicate to the group in character but as themselves when working with an individual resident who is confused or distressed. This duality gives them flexibility as artists but it also has physical and emotional consequences for them as people. How artists find strategies for looking after themselves when working in care homes is a question that is rarely considered, and it is important if care is to be conceived of as a reciprocal process.

In her book *The Managed Heart*, the sociologist Arlie Russell Hochschild introduces the concept of emotional labour to describe the process by which workers are expected to manage their feelings in accordance with organisationally defined rules and guidelines. She uses the example of flight attendants who are trained to continually smile in order to convey the 'right' feeling for the job, and subsequently, to induce the 'right' feeling in their passengers. This process, she suggests, involves 'individual acts of 'emotion work' and social 'feeling rules' (ix–x) which

> Require one to induce or supress feeling in order to sustain the outward countenance that produces the proper state of mind in others… This kind of labor calls for a coordination of mind and feeling, and it sometimes draws on a sense of self that we honor as deep and integral to our individuality. (Hochschild 2012, p. 7)

Hochschild is writing about emotion work in a very different context. By evoking her concept of emotional labour, I do not mean to suggest that artists working in care homes are required to induce or suppress certain feelings in order to convey the 'right' feeling to residents. However, her concept of 'social feeling rules' (ix) and the coordination of mind and feeling is instructive in understanding the sort of intuition that artists must draw on when leading a workshop in a care home. Hochschild associates emotional labour directly with the senses.

> I define feeling, like emotion, as a sense, like the sense of hearing or sight. In a general way, we experience it when bodily sensations are joined with what we see or imagine. Like the sense of hearing, emotion communicates information. (Ibid.: 17)

Her interpretation speaks to the emotional sensitivity and intuition that is required of artists as they decide how to proceed in a workshop. For example, at the beginning of the STORYBOX workshop, Sara and Lowri sensed that the appropriate thing to do in that moment was to join in with the activities that were happening in the room, rather than introduce their own. The decision about when to turn the TV down and put the music on also required them to work from intuition, since there was no formal beginning to the workshop. Hochschild's question' 'how does a person act on feeling?' (x) highlights the role of emotional intelligence and instinct in knowing how to proceed in this situation, particularly when attempting to find 'the sense of a beginning'.

These ideas on emotional labour have been advanced by the theatre scholar Erin Hurley in her book *Theatre and Feeling*, where she addresses the range of emotional experiences that are engendered by theatre. Considering the efforts of the actor, she suggests that the combination of physical and emotional work that is involved in performing convincingly, amounts to a type of 'feeling labour' (Hurley 2010, p. 38). Rather than seeing the emotional and physical effort as distinct types of labour, she describes this process as 'embodied emotional work' (ibid.: 64). This description is pertinent to the type of labour that is involved when facilitating in care homes. In particular, it speaks to the pressure that artists face from continually improvising and attuning to the activities of the room while still maintaining the forward direction of the workshop.

The notion of emotional labour in care homes has also been picked up by the theatre scholar Caoimhe McAvinchey. She describes the type of labour involved when artists work in care homes as a type of 'unusual labour' which requires 'a commitment of the artist to reveal something of herself' (McAvinchey 2013, p. 367), as well as negotiating a series of complex relationships with funders, care providers, residents and partner organisations. Reflecting on the work of Marysia Lachowicz, a visual artist who works in care homes, she describes a conversation in which Lachowicz revealed how much of herself she gave in her practice.

> You have to give quite a lot of yourself to get other people talking [...]. I build a rapport by sharing my life with people so they feel comfortable to share with me. I've brought in my photos, ones that I've taken, so it works as a two-way thing and they feel like they are getting to know me at the same time. (Ibid.: 367)

This account is consistent with the conversations that I had with the STORYBOX artists. Lowri told me that this process of continual improvisation could be extremely tiring as they felt that in order to do this successfully, she felt as if she were 'constantly performing'. The notion of emotional embodied work is a useful way of understanding the intuition that is required in this situation, and the emotional and physical consequences of this effort.

In Chapter two I used Kitwood's concept of giving and facilitation to suggest that reciprocity was a fundamental part of relationship-centred care. I suggested that the creative context of an arts workshop can increase the opportunities that people with dementia have to give in both a creative and caring capacity. Hochschild describes the way that people exchange gestures and feelings with each other as a 'gift exchange' in which 'each offers up feeling as a momentary contribution to the common good' (Hochschild 2012, p. 18). This analogy feels appropriate in understanding how people with dementia can care for artists in an environment where they are 'constantly performing'. In understanding the reciprocity that is involved in this type of care work, I am struck by a particular exercise that was led by the residents in the STORYBOX workshop. Each participant was offered their own balloon and invited to use it as a crystal ball which let them see into the future. As mystical music played, Lowri asked if anyone wanted to tell her fortune. The participants were receptive to her request. One of the residents said she was going to meet a tall handsome man. Another said that she would have seven beautiful children. Someone else piped up that she was going to live 'til she was 100'. There was something poignant about a group of women nearing the end of their lives predicting happy futures for the young women who were leading the workshop. After they had told Lowri's fortune the residents went on to tell each other's fortunes, predicting each other good health and long and happy lives. The exercise validated the status of people with dementia as skilled improvisers who could lead the facilitators in creative scenarios. Furthermore, it reflected their role as caregivers who were demonstrating a sort of 'fellow feeling' with the efforts of the artists. The residents in role as fortune tellers demonstrated the reciprocity of care-taking that takes place between artists and residents in a workshop. It emphasises the need for artists to experience care in a workshop and the role of residents as carers in an environment where they are primarily seen as recipients of care. Moreover, the fortune teller exercise demonstrated that the creative context of an arts workshop can increase opportunities for reciprocal acts of caregiving between artists and residents.

Embracing Slowness: 'The Social Aesthetics of Pace'

> Slow living involves the conscious negotiation of the differential temporalities which make up our everyday lives, deriving from a commitment to occupy time more attentively. Implicit in the practices of slow living is a particular conception of time, in which 'having time' for something means investing it with significance through attention and deliberation. To live slowly in this sense, then, means engaging in mindful rather than mindless practices which make us consider the pleasure or at least the purpose of each task to which we give our time. (Parkins 2004 p. 364)

In her article *Out of Time: Fast Subjects and Slow Culture*, the cultural theorist Wendy Parkins writes about the value and practice of 'slow living' in a late capitalist society, a process which she describes as paying mindful attention to everyday tasks. As the quotation suggests, slow living involves understanding the *differential* temporalities that make up everyday life and the reflection that is needed in order to live slowly. Parkins' work is instructive in understanding the value of slowness when doing arts practices in care homes and the way that artists attend to the differential temporalities of everyday life. The concept of slow living speaks to both the longer time frame that is needed for arts projects in care homes to take place and the quality of collaboration between an artist and an older person. Residents who have limited mobility or who are living with dementia may experience a different concept of time and speed to each other and to the artists who are working with them. Adopting the principles of slow living can encourage artists to embrace slowness in care settings, valuing the time that it takes for residents to arrive at and contribute to a workshop, and being mindful in how they engage with their contributions.

In her prologue to *Social Works*, Jackson cites the disability and performance scholar Petra Kuppers in order to consider the value of slowness as a 'new possibility for being in space' (Jackson 2011, p. 5). In *Disability and Contemporary Performance*, Kuppers analyses a passage written by Walter Benjamin which describes 'turtle-walking', a practice which was fashionable in early avant-garde arts practices, inspired by the idle walking practices of *flâneurs* in the 1840s. Kuppers considers the resonances of a turtle's pace slowing down its walker in light of what disability can offer to contemporary performance:

> Similar to the slow walk of the turtle walker disrupting the flow of the city, creating a different rhythm, the performances I investigate ... question ways of doing, ways of knowing as time slows or space expands... The turtle traverses an environment not built for short, stubby legs, its agency is in question, and yet it converses with the alien environment with every step it takes—no other option is open to it. In uneasy alignment, dialogues of being in space develop. Within the larger game plan of city life, turtle walking in the city is a minor, tactical insert into the systematic whole. (Kuppers 2003, p. 2)

When I first read this description it reminded me of care home resident Elena at Mildmay making a slow and determined beeline over to the sofa she wanted to sit on. Slow journeys such as these expose the production of spaces that take certain embodiments, such as mobility and speed, for granted. They also indicate the possibilities of care home residents in resisting the late capitalist desire for speed and efficiency. Older people can encourage artists to rethink the pace of their creative practice. According to Jackson, Kuppers' application of the 'social aesthetics of pace' in performance 'requires a change of internal odometer', a reconfiguration of pace which has the potential to 'engage our perception of wider social scales' and create a new 'dialogue of being in space' (ibid.: 5). By changing their internal odometer to fall in sync with the residents they are working with, artists may begin to embrace slowness as a quality or skill for working in care homes. In practice, this may include embracing the time it takes for those with limited mobility to arrive at a workshop, and accepting that people might arrive gradually over the course of a session. It may involve becoming more comfortable with taking time over a particular exercise, embracing slow and broken speech, allowing more time for people to speak, move or respond. It may involve accepting the repeated words and phrases of people with dementia, however many times they are said. In the example of STORYBOX, slowness also speaks to the time it takes for the workshop to start in negotiation with other activities in the care home. Jackson describes this as 're-calibrating ... objectives and the time it will take to reach them' (ibid.). Doing so, she suggests, may enable performance makers to register 'new possibilities for 'being in space' that had always been there' (ibid.). Her research suggests that artists and residents have the potential to creatively address the balance between slowness and fastness in a society which does not value those who move slowly.

In considering the social aesthetics of pace in a care home, it is also important to consider how time is experienced by residents in an environment where days may feel long and unstructured, or lacking in purpose. The cultural theorist Sarah Sharma suggests that understanding the value of slowness involves recognising 'how social experiences of time are multiple and uneven' (Sharma 2014, p. 111). For someone living with dementia, their experience of time may be very different to someone who hasn't experienced it. Similarly, for a resident who feels lonely and lacking in occupation, time may take on a different dimension to an artist who visits a care home on a weekly basis. Sharma argues that slowness can it be a strategy which enables people to maintain a distance from the temporal:

> Slowness appears to be about getting away, about maintaining distance from the temporal and the complex multiplicity of time. (Ibid.)

Embracing slowness in a care home not only involves acknowledging the time it takes for people to do things. It also involves understanding how the passage of time may be experienced differentially by people in care homes, particular if they are approaching the end of their lives or experiencing memory loss.

Finally, the concept of slow living also speaks to the burgeoning relationship that can develop between an artist and a care home, and the time that is needed in order for this to flourish. I had the opportunity to work with a care home over an 18-month period, getting to know staff and residents and allowing creative practice to develop gradually around the needs of the home. Valuing slowness as a way of working requires a funding culture which recognises the importance of long-term collaborations. This is particularly challenging in the current financial climate where there is a lack of sustainable funding for arts programmes is care homes. Artists and arts organisations relying on one-off project grants are often limited in the time scale of their delivery. In their *Arts in Care Homes* programme, Arts Council England stipulated that arts projects in residential care should be delivered over the course of three years in order to strengthen partnerships between care homes and arts organisations (Arts Council England 2013). This approach is important for a number of reasons. Long-term projects allow residents, staff and artists to get to know each other gradually, and for the creative work to be inspired by, and develop in response to, the care community. It also increases the opportunities for creative techniques being passed on to care staff, and for aspects of the creative work being integrated into the daily routines of the care home after a project has finished.

Note

1. See, for example, Oldham Coliseum Theatre, Theatre Royal Plymouth, and Royal Exchange Manchester.

References

Anderson, B., & Harrison, P. (2010). *Taking Place: Non-representational Theories and Geography*. Aldershot: Ashgate.

Arts Council England. (2013). *Arts and Older People in Care Commissioned Grant 2013: Guidance for Applicants*. Retrieved October 20, 2015, from http://www.artscouncil.org.uk/media/uploads/pdf/Arts_and_older_people_in_care_grant_guidance_notes.pdf.

Basting, A. (2001). God Is a Talking Horse. Dementia and the Performance of Self. *TDR, 45*(3), 78–94.

Cocker, S. (2014, November 11). Personal Communication with the Author.

Cohen-Cruz, J. (2010). *Engaging Performance: Theatre as Call and Response*. London: Routledge.

De Medeiros, K., Beall, E., Vozella, S., & Brandt, J. (2009). Television Viewing and People with Dementia Living in Long-Term Care: A Pilot Study. *Journal of Applied Gerontology, 28*(5), 638–648.

Forman, M. (2012). How We Feel the Music': Popular Music by Elders and for Elders. *Popular Music, 31*(2), 245–260.

Hallam, E., & Ingold, T. (Eds.). (2008). *Creativity and Cultural Improvisation*. London: Berg.

Harris, B. (2013). *The Storybox Project: Examining the Role of a Theatre and Arts-Based Intervention for People with Dementia*. Manchester: The University of Manchester.

Hochschild, A. (2012). *The Managed Heart: Commercialization of Human Feeling*. Berkley: University of California Press.

Hurley, E. (2010). *Feeling & Theatre*. London: Palgrave Macmillan.

Jackson, S. (2011). *Social Works: Performing Arts, Supporting Publics*. Oxon: Routledge.

Kraftl, P., & Horton, J. (2008). Spaces of Every-Night Life: For Geographies of Sleep, Sleeping and Sleepiness. *Progress in Human Geography, 32*, 509–524.

Kuppers, P. (2003). *Disability and Contemporary Performance: Bodies on the Edge*. Oxon: Routledge.

Lee, R. (2012). Interview with Martin Welton. *On Taking Care*. DVD. Arts Admin.

Leyser, M. (2012). Interview with Rosemary Lee. *On Taking Care*. DVD. Arts Admin.

Low, V. (2013, December 2). Plenty of Reasons to Laugh in this Loving, Happy Home. *The Times*. Retrieved December 20, 2014, from http://www.thetimes.co.uk/tto/public/timesappeal/article3937448.ece.

Mackley, K., & Pink, S. (2014). Moving, Making and Atmosphere: Routines of Homes as Sites for Mundane Improvisation. *Motilities, 11*(2), 1–17.

McAvinchey, C. (2013). Coming of Age: Arts Practice with Older People in Private and Domestic Spaces. *Research in Drama Education: The Journal of Applied Theatre and Performance, 18*(4), 359–373.

Parkins, W. (2004). Out of Time: Fast Subjects and Slow Living. *Time and Society, 13*(2–3), 362–382.

Peters, G. (2009). *The Philosophy of Improvisation*. Chicago: University of Chicago Press.

Sharma, S. (2014). *In the Meantime: Temporality and Cultural Politics*. London: Duke University Press.

Shin, J. S., Kim, M. S., Kim, G. H., Seo, S. W., Kim, E. J., Heilman, K. M., & Na, D. L. (2013). Excessive TV Watching in Patients with Frontotemporal Dementia. *Neurocase, 19*(5), 489–496.

Steger, B. (2003). Getting *Away* with Sleep: Social and Cultural Aspects of Dozing in Parliament. *Social Science Japan, 6*(2), 181–197.

Taylor, P. (2003). *Applied Theatre: Creating Transformative Encounters in the Community*. Portsmouth: Heinemann.

Welton, M. (2010). Listening-as-Touch: Paying Attention to Rosemary Lee's Common Dance. *Performance Research, 15*(3), 47–54.

CHAPTER 8

A Caring Effect

This chapter starts a process of identifying some longer-term effects of performance projects in care settings. Building on the relationship between creativity and care that I've outlined in previous chapters, it considers the effect that these sorts of collaborations can have on care settings. The effect of an arts project on a care home is not something that can be easily captured. Attempts to identify tangible 'outcomes' or 'impacts' that are attractive to funders are often complicated by the fact that participants may not remember taking part or may take part in a project at the end of their lives. Moreover, our understanding of the potential impact on a care home's working culture is limited if staff have been unable to participate in it.

Rather than looking to frameworks which attempt to measure change in quantifiable ways, my approach to understanding these types of effects is informed by questions of ephemerality in contemporary performance. In her book *Performing Remains*, theatre historian Rebecca Schneider uses the phrase 'performative trace' (Schneider 2011, p. 102) to describe what remains after a performance, and to challenge the archival desire to interpret performance relics as material documents. Drawing on the work of Jose Estaban Munoz, she contests the idea that ephemerality in performance is synonymous with disappearance. Instead, she contends that performance remains are 'distinctly material' in the 'traces, glimmers, residues and specks' (Ibid., p. 96) that remain after it has finished. Applied to a care setting, her theory offers a means of interpreting the more subtle affects

N. Hatton, *Performance and Dementia*,
https://doi.org/10.1007/978-3-030-51077-0_8

and shifts that can occur through creative practice. If I reflect on the end of my time with Mildmay, it is difficult to pinpoint changes that might be meaningful to those looking for quantifiable outcomes. However, I can identify some *affects* that emerged and continued to circulate after the work had finished. These were present in objects such as the envelope of magazine cuttings that resident Jean took to put in her scrapbook. And the colourful tablecloth that was bunched up by Rose, unseen by most, and slipped quietly into her handbag. A performative trace was made 'distinctly material' a few hours after our sound installation in the dining room when Elena, a resident living with dementia, quietly sang to herself the folk song we had learnt together. Such traces were also present in the atmosphere. When I visited Mildmay a week after our performance, a faint scent of flowers lingered in the dining room from the daffodils we had picked for the performance. These examples, though difficult to capture, are valuable to artists in articulating the subtle shifts that can occur through creative practice. As with an ecological approach to performance-making, understanding the 'remains' of a project involves identifying effects which occur at a microlevel.

The affective nature of these traces calls my phrase 'caring effect' into question. In using it, I am mindful of James Thompson's caution that concentrating on a performance project's *effects* on a community can reduce our appreciation of its purpose to identifiable social outcomes over aesthetic concerns. The performance practice and creative approaches to care discussed in this book are very much concerned with the 'terrain of sensation' (Thompson 2009, p. 117) and the 'capacity and intensity' (Ibid., p. 119) of affective bodies that he describes in his book *Performance Affects*. My use of the term 'effect' here is chiefly practical; a means of distinguishing between the affective processes at the heart of the practice and the broader, creative implications of the work. It is affectively attuned in the sense that it is concerned with the potential for subtle, microlevel shifts in working culture, and the performative traces that can be detected through an artist's practice in care homes to other projects. However, my interest in the longer-term implications of arts practices in care homes is also effect-*driven* in the sense that it is concerned with how wider economic factors are shaping how artists and care homes work together.

Working with Care Professionals: Supporting Differential Knowledge

Over the last decade, the scale and breadth of arts projects taking place in care homes has increased significantly. Many artists and companies have established approaches for working with older people in care homes and are now looking for ways of working with care professionals so that the creative practice may continue in some form after they have left. The challenge of involving carers in arts projects has been well documented by artists and funders, who acknowledge differences in organisational culture and the chaotic effect that artists can have on the routines of a care home. In their evaluation of the Arts Council's *Arts in Care Homes* programme, the Baring Foundation noted that 'experience of creative practice is not always a priority and the informal, improvisational and/or iterative approach of the artists can be viewed as disruptive or complex' (Dix et al. 2018, p. 19). Factors such as shift patterns can limit staff continuity across a project, as can high staff turnover and staff being sent to work across different sites. For many care homes, staff participation in an arts project is hampered by workload and the shifting, complex needs of residents. As one care home manager explained: 'People are coming into care at an older age now: they are less active with more health problems. It is an ever-changing, fluctuating environment… The duties of staff have changed as a consequence. The immediate, personal needs of residents are paramount and time consuming (Ibid., p. 9)'.

Taking part in creative activities is often additional work for care staff, particularly if it takes place outside of their contracted hours. When I attended a residents' cocktail party at Mildmay, I spent some time talking to a member of staff called Chloe who told me that she had worked a 14-hour shift in order to provide enough staff cover for the party to go ahead. I had volunteered to give manicures at this party and offered to give Chloe one too. She gladly accepted, but later got into trouble with her manager, who arrived towards the end of the party and wanted her to do the washing up as her nails were drying. In addition to highlighting the amount of work that takes place unnoticed in order to accommodate special events, the incident drew attention to the fact that participation in creative activities and special events can be perceived as a luxury.

In these circumstances it can be easy to overlook the knowledge and skills that care staff possess and the contribution that they can make to a creative process. The task-orientated nature of their workloads can mask the more creative attributes that we associate with good care, such as empathy, intuition and flexibility. Care staff may possess artistic talents, hold deep knowledge about the residents they care for, and about the internal politics and mechanisms of a care home. They may share a cultural heritage with a resident and be able to provide access to cultural reference points which shape and enrich creative practice. The task of bringing creativity into caregiving is a reciprocal process involving an exchange of differential knowledge. The skill of the artist is to find ways of eliciting the expertise of care staff and incorporating their specialist knowledge in the planning of creative projects.

In 2014 I worked as part of an evaluation team for a care home arts programme called *Hearts and Minds*, run by Age Exchange Theatre Trust in London. This project was for residents but a member of care staff was present at the workshops each week in order to assist with any physical care needs. Ongoing input from these carers was limited by the fact that there was usually a different member of staff attending each week. However, one of the researchers described how the cultural knowledge of care staff could still be used effectively in arts workshops, particularly when they were called upon for their expertise:

> Where expert knowledge about the residents' illness, condition and behaviour was shared, project workers were able to plan activities with greater understanding of how the work might be experienced and received. Where care staff were willing to participate in one-to-one activities or group work, the dynamic of the relationships between carer and resident changed, allowing the residents increased agency and creativity. Project workers were supported by care staff in practical ways, organising space and assisting with craft materials and creatively by ensuring that residents were able to continue their creative work between sessions. Care staff acted as 'cultural intermediaries' between residents and project workers. For example by explaining specific aspects of a resident's cultural background (life in the Caribbean, for example) or suggesting that a project worker's language skills might assist in communication with a resident with whose mother tongue was not English. (Nicholson et al. 2014, p. 75)

These observations suggest that unearthing the existing skills and knowledge of the care staff can enrich creative projects and strengthen relationships between artists, carers and residents. It is also an example of the social and cultural knowledge that carers can bring as 'intermediaries' between residents and artists. A further example of this can be found in the work of artist-researcher Jayne Lloyd, who has done cooking as part of her creative practice in care homes. On her website, Lloyd documents how she received help from the cook at the care home she was working with when making an ackee and saltfish dish with a resident. This Caribbean dish was native to the carer and the resident but Lloyd had never made it before. She was able to learn from both the cook and the resident when making the dish and to integrate their knowledge into her creative practice by making an illustrated cookbook based on their recipes.[1] Examples such as this indicate the value of getting to know care staff as well as residents in the planning stages of a project, in order to understand what skills and experiences they can bring to creative practice. They also point to the potential of embodied domestic activities such as cooking as an everyday creative practice that carers and residents can do together. Creating opportunities for residents to complete domestic tasks alongside carers may help to create a valued role for residents within the care community, as well as helping them to achieve a greater sense of home.

Embedded Practice

Inviting artists and residents into a care home kitchen is one example of how a care home routine, which takes up the majority of a staff member's time, may be approached in a creative way. In the same way that creative collaborations between artists and people with dementia involves improvisation, caregiving may also be seen as a creative and improvised process, rather than something which is repetitive and task-based. One of the evaluators for *Hearts and Minds* described the process of integrating creativity into caregiving as a type of 'embedded practice' (Ibid., p. 78). This phrase, which also appears in the Baring Foundation's evaluation of the Arts in Care Homes programme, is instructive in understanding how creative practice must be integrated broadly across the care home in different spaces, times and activities. In order for something to be 'embedded', it must be woven into the everyday fabric of the care home, across all acts of caregiving. The evaluator explains how embedded practice would work in an ideal situation:

> It takes place throughout the day and is not contained to a one hour arts and reminiscence session; It takes place in various locations throughout the care setting—it is not restricted to the activity room; it happens simultaneously or in conjunction with day to day care tasks—getting people up,

> washing, at meal times or whilst walking down the corridor, for example; it is delivered by someone native to the care setting rather than an outside agent; delivery becomes habitual or 'second nature'. (Ibid., p. 78)

The notion of creative practice that is habitual or second nature, and which takes place in conjunction with day-to-day care tasks, is important in shifting thinking away from care work as a task-based activity. In practice, it raises many questions, such as, what processes would need to happen in order for this practice to be adopted and become second nature? How plausible is it that a carer would have the time and energy to cultivate a new way of approaching their daily chores, in addition to getting through them? What support would need to be in place? How would we identify and acknowledge times when this is already happening and times when things could be done differently? Even with extensive training from artists, and supportive care home management, is difficult to imagine a situation where carers could find creative opportunities across all aspects of care giving. There are, however, some significant examples of carers integrating the techniques they have learnt during arts projects into primary care tasks. In her evaluation of STORYBOX, Bethan Harries noted that some of the carers who attended the storytelling workshops had started to identify connections between the creative activities they were learning and other aspects of care. In one care home, for example, 'a carer explained how she had taken a puppet with a patient to the toilet and demonstrated how the activities could feed into more mundane activities.' (Harris 2013, p. 56). Another carer remarked on how the physical nature of the drama workshops provided a creative means to incorporate exercise into the daily routine: 'Getting people moving their wrists and ankles in a creative way. We learnt about wrists and ankles in training and now I can see it being applied in this' (Ibid.). These examples point to the possibilities of integrating creative practice into the daily routines of caregiving and in particular, the physical and tactile aspects of care which can often be functional and impersonal. There is further scope to explore how creative techniques might be used during caregiving routines such as bathing, toileting and dressing, so that encounters between residents and caregivers become less functional.

Understanding embedded practice, I believe, also involves identifying the creative ways in which carers are already negotiating the competing demands of their workloads. While they might not immediately be interpreted as creative activities, I observed occasions at Mildmay where carers employed subtle forms of creativity to help them meet the needs of residents. There was a moment from the Old Film and Music Club which offered a good example of this. Though the care staff very rarely attended the sessions, there were a few occasions when a member of staff called Gloria was present. During the screenings, she would sit towards the back of the room and would often take the opportunity to catch up on her paperwork. At first, I interpreted this as a lack of engagement with the activities of the session. However, I watched in one session how she would sit at a table with two residents with dementia, holding one of their hands and moving it around in time to the music as she worked. There was something very natural and sociable about this small interaction and it seemed to be a rare opportunity for them to relax together. Furthermore, it showed how Gloria was skilfully paying attention to what was happening in the room while simultaneously continuing with a caregiving routine. This in itself was a form of creative practice which was distinct from any skill or exercise that could be taught by an artist.

Virtual Learning

While an embedded approach is a good idea in principle, it would most likely require artists to be working with or shadowing care staff over a considerable length of time in order to identify opportunities for creativity. Most creative partnerships with non-profit care homes are restricted by short-term project funding which limits their ability to cultivate these sorts of relationships. While there has been a huge increase in investment of the arts in care homes, the burden of financial responsibility for projects is still largely falling on the arts sector. Citing evidence from the All Party Parliamentary Group on Arts, Health and Wellbeing, the Baring Foundation identify that 'a time limited programme that provides a heavily subsidised intervention may have limited viability in the longer term, unless the changes it has brought about have affected strategic thinking and policy' (Dix et al. 2018, p. 40). In a climate of austerity where there is ongoing uncertainty about the future of the care sector, we are unlikely to see governmental investment in care home arts programmes anytime soon. The burden of funding is particularly acute for small arts organisations working in care homes who are often competing with venues that have subsidised programmes for older people. As Liz Postlethwaite, the creator of STORYBOX reflects, 'Arts and older people work is 'a different market now. There are arts organisations doing stuff for free which is actually really bad for people who need to make a living because people who live in a metropolitan urban setting get those things for free' (Postlethwaite 2019). The lack of financial support to develop projects with carers, coupled with the difficulties that carers face in finding time to take part, is encouraging some artists to think of new approaches.

Small Things' recently conceived 'arts by subscription' model, STORYBOX AT HOME, addresses some of the practical difficulties of implementing an embedded approach by creating a DIY package, where care homes subscribe to an archive of simple creative activities, tailored for individuals and groups. Subscribers are offered a one-day training workshop which introduces staff to Small Things' creative practice and encourages them to think about how they could replicate it in their setting. After this, care staff can access activities via a dedicated website in a way which fits around their routines. As Postlethwaite explains: 'The way that the website works is that subscribers every week get a full workshop plan with a theme. And then they get extension activities which are one the same theme. These can be stand-alone activities. They get a number of activities for groups and for individuals as well so if you're working with some people who are bed bound or not mobile... and what we try and encourage them to do is use the stuff within the context of the workshop but use it anywhere' (Ibid.).

As well as providing flexibility and ongoing support for carers who would like to try creative activities, this semi-commercial model means that the pressure of funding is more evenly distributed. It reduces the running costs to arts organisations while still enabling them to offer their expertise and creative tools to care staff as a product. The model is cost effective in that it's cheap for care homes (Small Things' subscription rate starts from £20 a month), but it has the potential to offer revenue to small arts organisations though building a portfolio of regular subscribers. So far, however, the evidence for care home take up of this scheme and similar ones is limited. We Do, one of the arts organisations funded through the Arts Council's Arts in Care Homes programme also piloted a semi-commercial approach where 'care homes signed up for an annual fee which included a free activity with training for care home staff and additional activities available to purchase at subsidised rates' (Dix et al. 2018, p. 16). The idea behind this pilot was to try and build sector demand and create a market for arts in care homes which was 'self-sustaining and economically viable' (Ibid., p. 2). Despite much promotion to care homes, few signed up and the programme was forced to close a year later. These examples indicate that there is more research to be done in order to understand the barriers and disincentives that are preventing care homes from accessing such programmes, as well as pursuing other options for sustainability.

An obvious limitation of a subscription approach is that it limits an artist's time in a care home. There is a risk that substituting artist residencies with a purchasable package of activities will promote an idea that arts practices are an approach that can be rolled out and delivered by anyone. This perception can diminish the purpose of professional arts practices in care homes and disincentivise policy makers from making meaningful investment. In the context of a social care funding crisis, a challenge for artists going forwards will be how they articulate the value of long-term partnerships with care homes and the unique skills that they bring. Simultaneously, in arguing for the creative role of the arts in care homes, there is a need to emphasise the ways in which artists foster a change in culture where the creativity of carers is nurtured and respected.

Carers as Performers: *Turning a Little Further*

> In a political situation in which care is both exceptionally necessary and exceptionally underprovided, acts of care begin to look politically radical. To care is to act against the grain of social and economic orthodoxy: to advocate care is, in the present moment, a kind of political rupture. (Giles 2016, p. 4)

The concluding part of the book departs from care homes and looks at carers in a different context in order to consider the effects that those with caring roles might have on contemporary performance more broadly. It considers what performance practitioners can learn from carers, and how they might shape their wider practice. Care is a subject which is currently commanding attention from performance scholars and practitioners who are exploring its application in a range of participatory and experimental performance settings. Jane Turner and Patrick Campbell's article *Radical Care* (2018), looks at generosity as a creative approach in the context of devising theatre with a transnational group of practitioners. A recently published book, *Performing Care* (2020), edited by Amanda Stuart-Fisher and James Thompson, explores the place of care in a range of socially-engaged performance contexts. Alongside this are a number of performances and community initiatives that are designed to engage the public in questions about care. *The Care Café*, instigated by performance artist Lois Weaver is a creative project which looks for 'ways to keep connected with each other in a real or virtual, public or domestic place' (Split Britches, n.d.). Alex Mermikides' experiential dance/theatre performance *Careful* (2016–) explores the interplay between performance and caregiving, putting its audience members in the role of patients in the care of five overstretched nurses. Developed in collaboration with nurses at Kingston University, the production initially invited nursing staff and students to be audience members and explored the difficulties of caring empathetically when struggling with exhaustion. The production simulates a hospital ward, with audience members reclined in beds, being visited and moved around by the actors. Over the course of the working day, the nurses become increasingly irritable and struggle to act compassionately. The physical routine of nursing is transformed into a dance routine which is repeated over and over with increasing speed until they fall out of sync and start to make mistakes. While the production represented, in one sense, an opportunity for nursing students to experience things from the perspective of their patients, it also raised disciplinary questions about what care means within a performance-making context.

What I'd like to explore in these final pages is what happens when those with caring responsibilities are placed at the centre of a performance process. This is in part a response to a question posed by Mermikides, about whether exposure to practices of care can 'allow performance practitioners to reconceive performance as a care-based discipline' (Mermikides 2016). Examining productions that feature carers as performers provides a particular insight into how values and practices that are associated with caregiving might be embedded within a performance process. Negotiating a devising process around caring responsibilities demands a way of working which departs from conventional rehearsal practices. Furthermore, having carers as writers and actors introduces new skills and experiences, which shapes the process in distinct ways. What I'm interested in articulating here is how collaborating with carers can generate distinctive approaches and modes of production. Furthermore, I am interested in the wider social function of these type of performances at a time where there is a massive breach between the need for care provision and the value that we place on it as a society.

My enquiry is influenced by Harry Josephine Giles' conception of care as a radical act, and in particular, their reflections on how to care for an audience. In their essay 'Shock and Care', Giles explores care as an avenue of artistic exploration, not so much a theme but a radical form which has the potential to disrupt. For Giles, care as an aesthetic choice is a radical alternative to more intrusive or uncomfortable forms of participatory performance that are designed to awaken, excite or disgust. They set out a series of strategies which explore what the 'art of care' might look like in a performance context, centring on different scenarios of audience participation. Examples of 'support structures that you can put around the artwork, to enable more people to better enjoy it' (Giles 2016) include

> allowing the audience to leave and return when they need to; providing space for interpretation and reflection; offering physical comfort to enable better engagement... [and] considering the accessibility of the language used in and around the artwork (Ibid.).

For Giles, these strategies aren't just fundamental to catering for diverse audiences. They offer a radical and necessary alternative to shows that are designed to shock their audience through discomfort. Caring for your audience in this way, they propose, has the potential to shock because it exposes the physical and emotional mechanisms of care in society where acts of care are invisible and undervalued. Giles' idea is instructive to performance practitioners who are working in care settings as it questions what this exposure to care can bring to performance making in other settings. This notion of 'care as shock' is an intriguing prospect for practitioners who are moving towards an understanding of participatory or applied performance which is care-led. Giles' suggestion that art which advocates care is a type of political rupture is an invitation to think about the radical potential of this type of performance, and how it might disturb the boundaries of what we considered to be shocking.

In 2015 the Young Vic Theatre in London staged *Turning a Little Further*, a production that was made with unpaid female carers and devised over several months around the cast's caring responsibilities. Though the context is different to the professional carers discussed in the rest of this book, it offers a rare insight into the qualities and insights that carers can bring to a rehearsal room. It is significant, not just because it deals with carers' experiences, but because of how negotiating caring responsibilities with the devising process necessitated a particular way of working. This approach departed from some of the conventions of creative production and offers some understanding of type of principles that might be associated with performances which are 'care-led'. By putting carers on the stage, *Turning a Little Further* also raises questions about theatre's capacity to change the status of carers in a society where the majority of caregiving is unpaid, undervalued and unseen.

Turning a Little Further was conceived by creative producer Lily Einhorn who worked on the theatre's Two Boroughs programme (now known as Neighbourhood Theatre). This long running project sees the theatre engage a community group from one of the neighbouring boroughs of Lambeth and Southwark and create a performance in response to the main house show. In this instance, Einhorn found herself seeking a group of women to work with alongside their production of Beckett's *Happy Days*. The Young Vic production featured Juliet Stevenson in the role of Winnie, the character who finds herself literally stuck up to her waist, and then up to her neck in sand. Reflecting on Einhorn's decision to approach a carers' group, director Laura Keefe thought it would be interesting to explore parallels between Winnie's predicament and women who felt 'that they were trapped in their everyday lives physically or mentally or that they themselves as carers found themselves trapped in places like their houses, the person that they cared fors' bedrooms, or that they mentally felt trapped' (Keefe 2019). The title of the carers' play, *Turning a Little Further* is a stage direction from Beckett's play, a reference perhaps to Winnies' constant attention to Willie and, as Einhorn explains, 'all those women, keeping the world turning, one day at a time' (Einhorn 2015). There is also, perhaps, a parallel to be made between the carers' situations and Beckett's reflections on the plight of the 'modern woman'. In 1994, the actress Brenda Bruce was interviewed about her experiences of working with Beckett and playing Winnie. She recounts Beckett's personal reflections on what was going through his mind when he wrote the play:

> Well I thought that the most dreadful thing that could happen to anybody, would be not to be allowed to sleep so that just as you're dropping off there'd be a 'Dong' and you'd have to keep awake; you're sinking into the ground alive and it's full of ants; and the sun is shining endlessly day and night and there is not a tree … there's no shade, nothing, and that bell wakes you up all the time and all you've got is a little parcel of things to see you through life… I thought who would cope with that and go down singing, only a woman. (Knowlson 1996, p. 501).

Comparably, Einhorn felt that their production was an opportunity to highlight the vital role of unpaid carers, who are predominantly women, and the 'often forgotten role [that they fulfil] in our society' (Einhorn 2015). The feeling of being 'up to your neck' was a motif that ran through the performance, through various personal stories, but unlike *Happy Days*, it was also a sincere celebration of their roles, their families, and their hopes for the future.

The production was performed in the Young Vic's Clare Studio by an intergenerational ensemble of 30 women. Fifteen of the performers were unpaid carers who had joined the project through local carers' 'hubs'—community organisations that offer support and respite to full time carers. Bringing together the company and devising a show around their caring responsibilities necessitated a more durational approach than previous Two Boroughs projects. It involved members of the Young Vic engagement team working at the hubs and getting to know potential participants gradually before inviting them to take part in the production. Initially, Keefe worked with the women over a 4-month period, meeting for two hours a week at the hubs. It was important to the producers that workshops were an opportunity for them to have some respite from their caring responsibilities first and foremost. The team ran exploratory workshops which gave the participants an opportunity to socialise, play games, and build confidence. For many of the participants, these two hours were the only time in the week that they had time to themselves. Moreover, the workshops provided a focus which was different from being a carer. As one performer, Jill Reyes, explained:

> It was something that was nothing to do with being a carer. It was something where I could express what I wanted to say. The role of a carer: what you feel, what you want to say isn't what you're dealing with. You don't have that opportunity, you are just focused on what this person needs now… you can't have a moment where you waiver. (Reyes 2019)

Once a company had been established, the creative team had to find some novel ways of addressing the difficulties of making a show on a heavily restricted schedule. Alongside the carer's groups, the Young Vic auditioned other women who lived in Lambeth and Southwark to be part of a core movement group. This 'shadow company' rehearsed more intensively alongside the workshops at the carers' hubs which addressed some of the difficulties of developing a production on a very restricted schedule. It enabled Keefe to spend more time crafting the initial material presented by the carers in movement sequences. Key routines were created during these sessions at the Young Vic and then taught to the carers during sessions at the hubs. Simultaneously, the show's writer, performance poet Francesca Beard, was working with the carers at the hubs on the development of a text. Once the participants had decided that they wanted to take part in the performance, creative material for the play was generated from these exercises at the hubs and woven together into a text by Beard. Personal aspects of individual caring stories were told by another performer in order to maintain anonymity and to ensure that the performers felt that their stories were being treated with care.

In an industry which is characterised by long hours and intensive periods of work, creating a supporting company or split roles might offer a new way of working for creatives with caring responsibilities. This opportunity is articulated by the theatre director, Caroline Wilkes who wrote in *The Stage* about her personal experiences of caring for two ill children while working as a theatre director. Wilkes reflects on the difficulties of directing part-time and how directors with caring responsibilities can seem like unappealing prospects to prospective theatres. The need for creative consistency, the long hours required when a show is in production can be seen as incompatible with the restrictions posed by medical appointments and 'crisis phone calls' during working hours. While acknowledging this difficulty, Wilkes challenges some of these 'norms' and poses some questions about how the theatre industry might adapt working practices in order to accommodate directors with caring responsibilities. One suggestion she poses, which is concurrent with the working practices in *Turning a Little Further*, is job sharing.

> I have worked with a smaller company where I have been able to direct in the mornings only and have the assistant director work in the afternoon with clear guidance. I have occasionally worked in a tag-team fashion as a director where, with very strong communication and trust built in, I have directed the first half of a week and my colleague directed the second half. (Wilkes 2018)

Wilkes is not offering a solution to the difficulty of working part-time on a show but a way of thinking about the options available to theatres who want to move towards inclusive working practices. While the success of a theatre production is often attributed to having creative consistency, these examples of shared creative roles support James Thompson's concepts of 'preparation and exhibition' in *Towards an Aesthetics of Care* where the 'supporting infrastructures of access are not the hidden mechanism of creative endeavour but a valued component of the aesthetics' which can 'demonstrate and model a form of mutual regard' (Thompson 2015, p. 438). Creative examples of supporting or caring infrastructures run throughout this book, from dramaturgical scaffolds that support the participation of people with dementia as theatre-goers, to the distributive agency that can occur between people and things during workshops in care homes, and the way in which Lee's performers looked after each other in *Common Dance*. In the context of the theatre industry, however, the needs of professionals who are carers are often invisible or perceived to be incompatible with any sort of creative process. Putting carers on stage is one way of challenging these working practices as it simultaneously informs and establishes a supportive aesthetic which is unapologetic in its presentation of support mechanisms.

While negotiating a rehearsal process around caring responsibilities required an adaptive way of working, one thing that emerged from the production is how some of the qualities associated with caregiving were particularly suited to a theatre-making process. One of the performers I spoke to, Boma Braide, drew a connection between her caring and performing roles, reflecting on how being a carer required her to perform a series of acts that were repeated in way that was comparable to the process of repeating a performing on stage each night. 'It's an action, isn't it. There is a link. When you are caring you a doing an act. Not an act, but a routine, a type of thing you do. You're performing a routine, you follow a pattern. Caring is a pattern' (Braide 2019). Jill Reyes spoke of how her 'ability to cope with anything and everything' had equipped her with the confidence to improvise if something went wrong on stage, and likened the 'sheer physical stamina' required for caring for her husband with the physical endurance of performing on stage every night (Reyes 2019). This combination of extreme physical and emotional endurance is picked up by Caroline Wilkes' in her reflections on her own role as a director-carer. Her reflections on the transferability of caring roles to the rehearsal room are novel and worth quoting in full:

> Carers often have a depth of understanding and insight born out of managing endless, complicated situations. Such understanding can bring significant human insight and fresh perspectives into the rehearsal room. From a

> pragmatic perspective, being a carer equips someone with skills that are relevant to the theatre. Whether juggling multiple demands simultaneously, the patience needed, the privilege of experiencing the world from a very different perspective or fighting for provision, caring provides huge insight into human nature at its most raw. Then there is the tact and diplomacy needed, being able to keep your eye on the many small details as well as the larger ones, the endless problem solving, thinking on your feet, dealing with conflict, being strong at both written and verbal communication (and the importance of being a strong listener) and sheer dogged resilience. It also gives us a deep sense of perspective about life with all its fragilities. (Wilkes 2018)

Wilkes' parallel between care and the rehearsal room raise questions about the values that the theatre industry places on carers, and the relevant experience that they bring to any production process, regardless of what the show is about. In terms of my enquiry, they also raise questions about the type of creative process that is most conducive to representing the experiences of carers on stage. The Young Vic's production was an example of how caring attributes can be embedded in process and product. In a similar way to how care was both a 'mode and a matter' of performance in *Common Dance*, care became a theme and a way of working in *Turning a Little Further*. The need to provide a respite environment had a creative influence on devising as well as inspiring the dynamic of the sessions at the hubs. A question, 'where do you go to escape, either as a physical place or in your mind?' was posed early on in the process as a way of encouraging the participants to think about their lives outside of their caring roles. Many of the participants mentioned the role of music in their lives as something that helped them to escape or feel strong during difficult times. Prompted by this discovery, the facilitators invited them to bring along a piece of music that was important to them and to tell the story of the song's significance to the rest of the group. These stories about music embedded themselves in the performance text in the form of snapshots, illustrating different moments in the carers' lives:

> **Maria**: I listen to music, a song of the moon floating above the sea, The swaying melody, lilting movements as the waves meet the shore, the coast breeze, with the blue shining above, this takes me back to memories, to happiness…. (Beard 2015, p. 6)

Kemi: ......And when I hear this song, I see my daughter, dancing on her fourth birthday, dancing with such abandon, singing out loud, eyes closed, flinging her little body around.... (Ibid., p. 5)

These lines are indicative of the poetic imagery that characterises much of the play, particularly when voices are capturing moments that take place outside of their caring responsibilities. However, the text is also direct in its treatment of care as a physical and repetitive experience. It weaves together some of the rhythms and pulls of caregiving in an abstract style with some more literal examples from the carers' experiences. As one of the performers, Hilary Friend, explained: 'it was this nice combination of quite expressive, almost abstract material with the words with these very real, very direct illustrations of real experience' (Friend 2019). There are moments where the punctuated rhythm of the text mirrors the experience of being overloaded:

Nicole: Time.
Joanna: An hour –
Deborah: Half –
Penny: A quarter –
Elanor: Five –
Kemi: Two –
Malinda: One –
Doreen: Minute –
Maria: Give me just a –
Andi: Just give me a –
Posy: Second
Turn
Again (Beard 2015, pp. 1–2).

At other moments, the text draws attention to caring attributes in a more open, poetic form. The words that open the play are celebratory, a validation of carers' roles, and a call to action:

Rise up Women,
Whose name means Caring, Strength, Hope, Beauty,
Begin again, another happy day (Ibid.).

Though the development of a text and the collaboration with Beard were a fundamental part of the performance, the company chose not to produce a dramatic script with identifiable characters. Instead, a text was created which prioritised 'movement throughout and the dialogue would go over the top' (Keefe 2019). This decision opened up a space to explore some of the physical and sensory aspects of caregiving, which was supported by the ongoing input of a movement director—Coral Messam. The decision to tell their story through movement as much as text was in part a deliberate departure from the static nature of *Happy Days* but it also provided an opportunity to build practices of care into the devising process. For example, the question was posed: 'how do you feel when you get a moment to yourself'? Participants were invited to explore that feeling physically with the instruction: 'Can you express that with a word, can your express that with a sound, and then can you express that with a movement' (Ibid.). This sequence was used as a base to develop more expansive movement sequences, alongside routines which were based on the daily routines of caregiving. As Keefe explains: 'we'd go through the day physically and distilled that into something more abstract. One sequence that was about caring: I think it was a group of 3. It started as an exercise where they had to maintain contact or like 'over and under' so they had to keep moving around' (Ibid.). Like Mermikides' production *Careful*, the choice to start with movement enabled the physical and feeling aspects of care to be experienced rather than intellectualised through a narrative. These physical sequences also provided an opportunity for participants to stretch out their bodies and move them in ways that were not part of the physical routine of caring. (Keefe noted that some of the women had back problems as a consequence of caring and didn't have many opportunities to exercise or stretch out their muscles).

Alongside these performance choices, working with carers as performers encouraged the company to think about ways in which practices of care might be embedded across production elements. As none of the women had performed before, Keefe's priority was to make them feel as safe as possible as well as creating a caring aesthetic for the audience. The set provided an enclosed, intimate space for the performers with soft textures, rather than the feeling of a bare floor underfoot. As Keefe explains

> The audience sat around them and the set was memory foam mattresses. The idea was that it would feel a bit like a bed… And there was a canopy over them which was a sheet, so like a bedsheet, but when you lifted it up it could create clouds, we put lights behind it so it could create rainbows. It all felt… there was a constant soundscape that had a womb heartbeat and the sound of the sea' (Ibid.).

This environment was emphasised through directorial choices which saw the performers remain on stage throughout and much of the stage action being played inwardly to each other rather than to the audience. A notable moment comes at the end of the play where the performers dance and throw gold confetti. This sequence takes places with the performers facing each other in a circle rather than out to the audience. This decision to put the performer's welfare ahead of the audience experience disrupts a theatrical convention but it is concurrent with Thompson's definition of exhibition, which prioritises the interdependent nature of a performance outcome over 'a display of singular creative expertise or virtuosity' (Thompson 2015, p. 439). As he suggests, 'this form of cooperation might involve a challenge to the quality and texture of a rehearsal or devising experience so that the reciprocity of gradual creation is valued over and above the discipline of the single-minded voyage towards the first night' (Ibid., p. 438) (Fig. 8.1).

In thinking through what it means in practice to 'perform care', *Turning a Little Further* provides some orientation for those engaged in

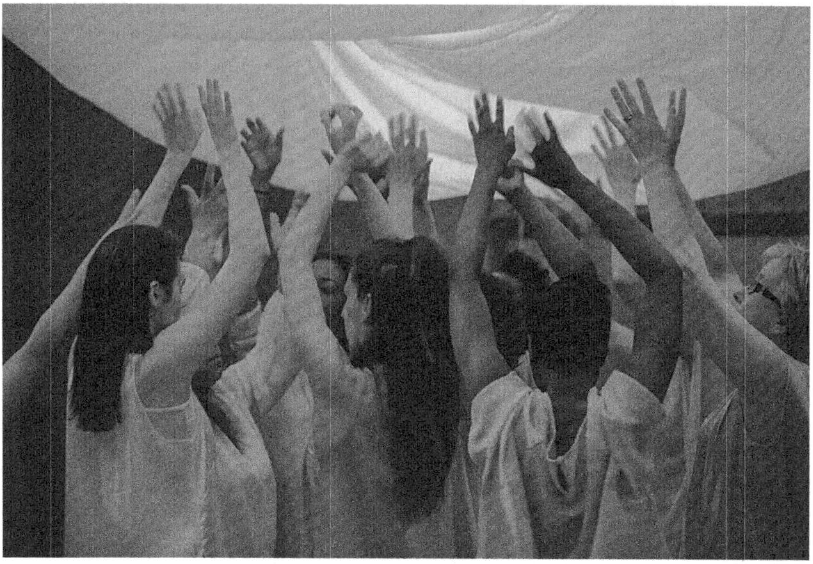

Fig. 8.1 *Turning a Little Further*. The Young Vic Theatre, 2015. (Photograph by Helen Murray)

community performance as to how practices of care can be traced from private process through to public outcome. What is distinct about this production compared to other examples of socially engaged performance is that the expertise of the women *as carers* was utilised in the development of the show and woven into its creative material. At times, the performance struck a maternal tone where the local knowledge and wisdom of the women formed the basis of interactions with the audience. In a tongue-in cheek section of the play, the carers dispensed advice to 'women of 2015' in the form of a 'guide to life'. Delivered in direct address, this section offered suggestions which ranged from the practical and playful to the more profound:

> Get a properly fitted bra…
> Do pelvic floor exercises at the bus stop…
> Take part in the struggle to build a better world—it is women and children who suffer most in an uncaring society…
> Encourage younger women—The world finds it easy to ignore their promise (Beard 2015, p. 9).

Without the context of the play, this invitation to care for oneself may have rung hollow, particularly in the light of the growing commercialisation of 'selfcare'. What distinguished the invitation made by the performers is that they care for people 24 hours a day. It highlights a curious breach between our occupation with self-care and the value we place on the carers in our communities. The visibility of the self-care industry across so many areas of our lives feels rather at odds with the invisibility of carers and their status in our society—what journalist Madeline Bunting articulates as a 'systematic cultural and historical undervaluing of care… and a profound lack of respect for the labour of care' (Bunting 2016).

While there are moments in the play which address the difficulties of being a carer up front, care is more the form of the performance than the theme. This is apparent in the ways that the performers care for each other and the audience, and in the various ways that the show explores the feeling and sensory aspects of care. By avoiding a dramatic narrative about carers in crisis, the show challenged the stereotype of care as a low skilled and undesirable occupation. Instead, it made visible the type of positive attributes that are associated with care, positioning the performers as skilled experts. The potential of this type of performance to elevate the status of carers was identified by performer Hilary Friend who reflected that: 'It released a feeling of feeling quite important' (Friend 2019). Shows that look after performers and audiences in this way remind us what it feels like to be cared for and give us pause to reflect on our own caring roles. They also have the potential to change the way in which theatre directors approach any sort of theatre project. When I asked Keefe how the production had shaped her as a director, she spoke of how it had given her an increased awareness of the role of care within a performance-making process, regardless of who the company are:

> It made me more conscious, and this is something that is in my practice now, of checking in with people and knowing that people are going to be bringing stuff in the room with them and hopefully not leaving with that... And how to treat an audience. Sometimes when I do professional work it's been quite autobiographical, sometimes it deals with issues that can be quite emotional so it made me think about looking after myself and the performers and looking after the audience as well. (Keefe 2019)

By putting those with caring responsibilities at the centre of a performance process, productions such as *Turning a Little Further* expand our understanding of conventional production processes. This is not to overlook the challenges of creating consistency when accommodating part-time roles, but similarly to a dramaturgy of assistance, it offers a different way of thinking about the journey of creative production. There is an ongoing need to rethink working practices to make it possible for those with caring responsibilities to continue with creative roles. This will enrich the theatre industry, opening it up to knowledge and experiences that are fundamental to creative thinking and the sharing of human experience. Shows which deal with care explicitly as a theme or a mode helps us to articulate the shape and feel of care at a time when it is needed most. With a social care sector that has now exhausted its capacity for further cuts, we need more public narratives that advocate for care, and which prioritise caring attributes above speed, efficiency and independence. Theatre about care encourages us to broach urgent, uncomfortable conversations about ageing and capacity. It helps to normalise care as a visible and essential component of an ageing society, rather than an undesirable inconvenience which is the private burden of families. Shows such as *Turning a Little Further* push us to think about how we would like to be cared for in the future and argue for interdependence as a viable option.

The possibilities of care as a performative concern are still emerging. Perhaps what represents the most intriguing prospect for me is how a new generation of performance makers will respond to these concerns as they fight to stay afloat in an increasingly precarious, neoliberal environment. When negotiating overinflated rents, internship cultures, and transactional models of Higher Education, the lure of #selfcare as a survival mechanism is understandable. What remains to be unearthed is the point at which this deeply individualised philosophy starts to feel incompatible with working as an artist. As a theatre lecturer, there is a question for me about how care may be embedded in the way we teach performance practice in universities. Giles' proposition, 'how we can positively, creatively and with deep meaning care for the audience?' (Giles 2016), feels pertinent to those teaching performance in Higher Education, many of whom are currently fighting to justify its place within a marketplace system.

While writing this chapter I came across an independent verbatim theatre company—Ecoute Theatre which is run by young women. It currently has two shows in production—*Take Care*, which focuses on the 'human story behind end-of life-care' and *Risk Assessment*, which 'explores the dangerous moral and ethical consequences of treating students as customers' (Ecoute Theatre 2019). Are these two productions connected? That these millennial performance makers cared enough to make these shows, and in tandem, suggests that they are questioning the consequences of this culture of independence on their own futures. For artists that are involved in verbatim processes, the idea of approaching theatre making with a caring frame feels especially relevant.

Another example of young people making theatre within a caring frame is visible within the undergraduate Drama programme that I work on at York St John University. In a second-year module, we invite students to 'plan, design, scale and implement a small scale politically engaged piece of arts activism' (Reason 2018, p. 2), connected to an issue which matters to them. While many of our students do not identify with conventional definitions of activism or activists, the notion of 'quiet activism' as a practice which includes 'small, quotidian acts of kindness, connection and creativity' (Pottinger 2017, p. 215) is an idea which resonates with many of them. An aesthetic of care, kindness, and interdependence has shaped many of these activist projects, as well as their work on other modules. One group of students, inspired by Yoko Ono's 1966 installation *Mend Piece*, invited people on campus to join in with mending broken teacups, as a metaphor for mental health and fragility. Another group created a project called *The Sofa Experiment*, where they took a sofa around the centre of York and 'invited the public to sit… have a cup of tea, a slice of cake and tell us something interesting about them' (Three Sides Theatre 2011). In a climate where an increasing number of students are experiencing mental health issues, these projects show how students can engage with care as a critical and creative concern across different types of performance practice. The strategies of care discussed throughout this book: slowing down, attuning, interdependency, and paying attention to the more-than-human, might be tools that a new generation of performance makers can embed within their work, as a means of counteracting the more damaging implications of selfcare culture.

Note

1. A Taste of Life' is available for download from Lloyd's website: https://www.jaynelloydart.com/copy-of-luggage-1.

References

Beard, F. (2015). *Turning a Little Further.* (unpublished). The Young Vic Theatre.

Bunting, M. (2016). *Crisis of Care. The Essay. BBC Radio 3.* Recorded at The British Academy on 11th February 2016. https://www.bbc.co.uk/programmes/b0741jl8. Accessed online 23 August 2019.

Dix, A., Gregory, T., & Harris, J. (2018). *Each Breath is Valuable: An Evaluation of an Arts in Care Homes Programme.* Baring Foundation. Retrieved August 23, 2019, from https://cdn.baringfoundation.org.uk/wp-content/uploads/Each-breath-is-valuable_arts-in-care-homes-FINAL.pdf

Ecoute Theatre. (2019). Retrieved August 24, 2019, from https://www.ecoutetheatrecompany.com/our-shows

Einhorn, L. (2015, May 12). Turning a Little Further—Two Boroughs at the Young Vic. Retrieved August 23, 2019, from https://youngviclondon.wordpress.com/2015/05/12/turning-a-little-further-two-boroughs-at-the-young-vic/

Giles, H.. (2016). Shock and Care. Retrieved August 23, 2019, from https://harryjosephine.com/2016/04/24/shock-and-care/

Harris, B. (2013). The Storybox Project: Examining the Role of a Theatre and Arts-based Intervention for People with Dementia. Manchester: The University of Manchester.

Knowlson, J. (1996). *Damned to Fame: The Life of Samuel Beckett.* London: Bloomsbury.

Mermikides, A. (2016, December 15). *Performance, Nursing and the Embodiment of Care*. Unpublished conference paper, Performing Care Symposium, The Royal Central School of Speech and Drama.
Nicholson, H., Handler, S., Johnson, R., Hatton, N., Lloyd, J., & Sears, R. (2014). Summative Evaluation of Hearts and Minds. A Three-Year Pilot Programme by Age Exchange Theatre Trust. Royal Holloway, University of London. Retrieved December 30, 2015, from http://www.eyesociation.org/AgeExchange/SummativeEvaluationHeartsandMinds.pdf
Pottinger, L. (2017). Planting the Seeds of a Quiet Activism. *Area, 49*(2), 215–222.
Reason, M. (2018). Students as Arts Activists: Insights and Analysis from a Politically Engaged Assessment. *Arts Praxis, 5*, 2–17.
Schneider, R. (2011). *Performing Remains: Art and War in Times of Theatrical Reenactment*. London: Routledge.
Split Britches. (n.d.). Retrieved August 23, 2019, from http://www.split-britches.com/care-cafe
Stuart-Fischer, A., & Thompson, J. (Eds.). (2020). *Performing Care: New Perspectives on Socially Engaged Performance*. Manchester: Manchester University Press.
Thompson, J. (2009). Performance Affects. *Applied Theatre and the End of Effect*. Basingstoke: Palgrave Macmillan.
Thompson, J. (2015). Towards an Aesthetics of Care. *Research in Drama Education, 20*(5), 430–441.
Three Sides Theatre. (2011). *The Sofa Experiment*. Retrieved February 26, 2020, from https://www.youtube.com/watch?v=Aet39UERDkY
Turner, J., & Campbell, P. (2018). Radical Care. *Performance Research, 23*(6), 58–65.
Wilkes, C. (2018, November 18). It's Time to Change Theatre's Working Practices to Support Carers. *The Stage*. Retrieved August 24, 2019, from https://www.thestage.co.uk/opinion/2018/director-caroline-wilkes-its-time-to-change-theatres-working-practices-to-support-carers/

Interviews/Correspondence

Braide, B. (Performer). (2019, July 17). *Turning a Little Further. Interview*, Bradford.
Friend, H. (Performer). (2019, April 30). *Turning a Little Further. Interview*, Bradford.
Keefe, L. (Director). (2019, May 6). *Turning a Little Further. Interview*, Bradford.
Postlethwaite, L. (Director). (2019, February 4). Small Things Creative Projects. *Interview*, Manchester.
Reyes, G. (Performer). (2019, May 1). *Turning a Little Further. Interview*, Bradford.

CHAPTER 9

Conclusion

The task I set myself with writing this book was to offer some new ways of thinking about dementia care, and to understand what performance might offer in supporting it as a creative endeavour. I began with a premise that transformation was the wrong goal and that there had to be a way of working with care homes as individual places rather than institutions. By taking the environmental and communitarian qualities of a care home as a starting point, I have endeavoured to show how artists can move towards a more symbiotic relationship with them. In many ways, this type of responsiveness is a hallmark of any good creative partnership, but the argument presented here is that there is something particular to be learnt from care homes about building from the centre-outwards.

Early on in *Social Works*, Shannon Jackson critiques the idea of 'artist-as-community-helpmate' (Jackson 2011, p. 44), suggesting that there may be other 'critical barometers' with which to evaluate the relationship between an artist and a community group. This is not because she is opposed to definitions of social art that are community-focused but because helpmate models, in addition to implying a unidirectional relationship of support, may rely on a limited concept of community. 'To what does a term like community refer?' she asks. 'Does it pursue or enforce visons of harmony and consensus?' (Ibid.). Care homes also trouble certain ideas of community. The convergence of communal and private spaces, the juxtaposition of home and work, and the presence of structured routines require artists to fall into step with an unfamiliar system.

N. Hatton, *Performance and Dementia*,
https://doi.org/10.1007/978-3-030-51077-0_9

Jackson's barometer is an appropriate metaphor for a more ecological approach to performance-making which seeks to respond to the unique climate of a care home; a climate which may not immediately seem conducive to making performance. This is not to suggest that all challenges can be turned into opportunities. There are some very real incompatibilities between the arts and care sectors that cannot be overcome by simply paying attention to a care environment or employing sensory approaches. The delicate skill of the artist in this situation is to remain alert to the creative possibilities of a care home, which may not be obvious, while also incorporating their specialist knowledge and introducing new possibilities for the space.

Performance and Dementia makes two key arguments. The first, outlined in detail in Chap. 4, is that any notion of relationality in dementia care must account for the relationships that people with dementia have with the non-human. A key focus was defining a relational approach to care which was inspired by posthuman notions of distributive agency and, following Jane Bennett, the vibrancy of matter. In the context of a care home, this sort of matter includes material and atmospheric features such as sounds, objects, and spatial arrangements which can be powerful institutional signifiers but can also help people with dementia navigate a care home. In some cases, these familiar or appropriated objects can facilitate participation in the social life of the care home or help residents to avoid it. Seeing, or feeling, the material environment of a care home as creative terrain opens up opportunities for sensory and experiential encounters which in turn help us to understand dementia care as a more-than-human interaction.

The practice-based discussion in Chap. 5 explored a specific manifestation of vibrant matter in a dementia care context. Working with sound opened our sensibilities, as performance practitioners, towards the ways in which cares spaces are heavily constituted by sound, but also how sound could connect to other times and places that were significant to the residents. Sound was a sensory reference point for these participants because it always associated itself with a place, whether it was a place in the care home or somewhere entirely different. To revisit the idea of sound theorist Brandon LaBelle, the sounds that were explored 'simultaneously embed[ded] us with local environments' while also 'connecting us to a broader horizon' (2006, p. xii). The practices of listening that characterised the project, and the idea of bodies interpreting the sounds and making them resonant, positioned listening as a place-making activity. It is an example of how the agency of place-making was distributed between human bodies and non-human sounds, rather than something that was institutionally imposed.

By analysing performance work which explores relationships between people and things, I have tried to provide some insight into what a relational approach to dementia care might look like in practice. My attempt to flesh out the components of this approach through a performance lens comes at a time where scholars from other disciplines are also beginning to explore the possibilities of the arts in supporting relationality in dementia care. Pia Kontos, for example, has conducted a mixed method study which explores the role of elder clowns in 'advanc[ing] a model of relational citizenship for people with dementia' (Kontos et al. 2017, p. 182). As questions of interdependence, citizenship and reciprocity are starting to shape thinking and practice, I hope that this interpretation of dementia care as a posthuman endeavour will contribute to these wider conversations, as well as providing some orientation for artists who are working with people with dementia inside and outside of care settings.

The second argument made in *Performance and Dementia* is that the arts have a cultural role to play in supporting dementia care as a creative practice. Pinning down what a 'cultural response' means in the context of the field of arts and dementia required me to look specifically at notions of value in arts and health research, and to find ways of articulating changes that are subtle, affective, and not always replicable. In Chap. 2, the call for a cultural response was set against the cultural construction of dementia in the West as a tragedy which equates to a 'loss of self'. This book questioned the prominence of the self as an autonomous figure which is maintained through active economic participation in society. Much of this critique was centred on the predominance of wellbeing in the field of arts and health which often places the responsibility of being well with the individual and assumes a level of capacity and conformity. The practice explored in this book exposes wellbeing as an inadequate mantra and justification for arts in dementia care in and of itself. One of the benefits of placing artists in care homes is that their practice can validate a range of emotional experiences and states of wellness. Magic Me, the intergenerational charity who ran an artist residency programme in care homes identified this as a key learning point for the artists who worked on it: 'Artists were keen to keep activities happy and upbeat but over the course of their work they learnt that it was actually a good thing to create space for deeper emotional reactions and experiences through the art forms' (Begault et al.

2017, p. 31). Similarly, one of the most palpable skills demonstrated by artists Lowri Evans and Sara Cocker during the STORYBOX workshop was how they responded carefully to the solemn atmosphere in the room on Remembrance Day without trying to cheer everybody up.

In advocating for the creative role of performance in dementia care, this book is not trying to overlook the very well documented health benefits of participation. There is a balance to be struck in continuing to understand and promote the health benefits of the work while finding ways to articulate the value of arts in dementia care in its broadest sense. Rather than contesting arts and health research that looks for measurable changes and outcomes, my hope is that this book will deepen conversations about value and artistry and offer some responses to the challenges of cross-sector collaboration.

An important theme in this book is the way that residents negotiate the social environment of a care home and how an arts project intersects with the politics of space and the impositions of communal living. In Chap. 6, a connection was revealed between the nature of participation in an arts project and participation in the social life of the home. In a situation where residents have limited opportunities to express personal tastes or preferences about who they spend time with, sensory arts practices can nurture attachments to objects, spaces and places as well as revealing commonalities between residents. Pop music was revealed to be particularly significant in highlighting commonalities and divergences in taste, and how factors such as ethnicity, age, and socioeconomic backgrounds can shape the way that residents signal their identity to others. This practice also challenged some common assumptions about taste in later life; the idea that older people will always enjoy the music from their youth, and the assumption that people from the same generation will like the same sort of music. Research into the significance of musical taste in later life is still emerging and the work of gerontologists such as Murray Forman and Andy Bennett suggests that there is more to be done in order to understand the sociocultural significance of music for people living in care homes.

Part of understanding the cultural role of the artist in dementia care involved cultivating an awareness of the connections between creativity and care and the contribution that carers and people make to an artistic process. While it can be difficult for carers to take part in arts sessions, identifying carers as cultural intermediaries who have specialist knowledge about residents can allow them to contribute in different ways, and at different stages of a partnership. By offering some examples of how carers are integrating creative techniques into their work, this book has advanced the idea of embedded practice as something which takes place routinely, between residents and carers, without the presence of an artist. Embedded practice requires an attunement on behalf of the artists towards the many ways that carers already demonstrate creativity within the competing demands of caring roles. These forms of creative practice may share attributes with an artist's creative practice such as improvisation, resourcefulness and resilience. In the same way that artists must attune to the 'everyday creativity' demonstrated by care homes residents, working with carers requires an appreciation of different types of creativity, and how the differential knowledge of artists and carers is essential to a successful partnership.

In understanding the particular role of theatre and performance in dementia care settings, this book has been influenced by performance makers who are exploring dementia outside of care homes. Chapter 3 traced a cultural shift in representations of dementia on the British stage from plays about dementia and caregiver burden, towards a theatre of co-creation. For Melanie Wilson and Platform 4, the process of collaborating with people with dementia fostered an experiential approach which simulated the lived experience of dementia and foregrounded the role of the sensory world in how people with dementia make sense of their environment. By closely examining the processes involved in making dementia-friendly theatre, this book has endeavoured to offer new insights into access as an aesthetic choice as well as an inclusive practice. The dramaturgical possibilities of dementia-friendly theatre were extracted through an exploration of *Every Third Minute* festival, which embedded strategies of interdependence across different stages of creative production. Examples of interdependence were discernible across the programming process, which asked artists to think differently about how they communicated their ideas. It was present in the concept of a 'generous audience', in the technical adaptations made to productions in order to create a more comfortable sensory experience for audiences, and in the development of the scratch performance night, which gave a platform to artists who were living with dementia. These strategies increased the accessibility of the performances but also raised wider questions about the relationship between performance and participation. The practice of bringing together an intergenerational audience for a dementia-friendly performance, for example, offers a new way of looking at the experience of theatre-going as a state of shared vulnerability where the needs of each audience member and performer is accepted, and everyone plays a role in creating a supportive environment. As more theatres are starting to put neurodiversity on their programming agendas, offering residencies for neurodiverse artists, exploring relationships between neurodiverse characters, and casting neurodiverse actors in shows about their experiences,[1] these creative scaffolds may become familiar features in mainstream theatres. Rather than looking at these choices as adaptations for a minority audience, the features of dementia-friendly theatre may be interpreted, as Matt Hargrave suggests, as a 'full[er] range of aesthetic forms in order to tell the stories that most matter' (Hargrave 2017, p. 228).

What began as a book about care homes concluded by exploring broader connections between care and contemporary performance. In the final two chapters, parallels were drawn between the qualities of collaboration in a theatre and dementia project and performance artists for whom care is both a mode and a theme in their practice. Intertwining an analysis of the STORYBOX project with Rosemary Lee's work enabled me to create a methodology for collaborative performance-making based on practices of attention and attunement. Similarly, the creative scaffolds displayed during *Every Third Minute* feel in some ways connected to the support mechanisms that characterised the devising process in *Turning a Little Further*—a production which skilfully placed carers at the centre of a creative process. A distinction was drawn between the generative practices of care that went into this production and a growing neoliberal trend towards self-care as a market and lifestyle practice. By making time for a lengthy devising process, forming a shadow company and creating a text which simultaneously celebrated the role of unpaid carers and articulated the physical and emotional impact of being overloaded, the play demonstrated how caring attributes can be woven across process and product. Following Giles' description of 'radical care', performances such as this may productively challenge the tendencies of radical performance towards discomfort and disturbance as well as countering a more damaging culture of '#selfcare'.

As arts practices in dementia care grow and expand, and the landscape of our care sector shifts, many of the ideas offered here will be transformed and challenged through future practice. I hope that the possibilities of performance as a mode of care and care as a mode of performance will continue to be interrogated. While the shape and feel of care can manifest in different creative ways, each of the performances explored in this book, regardless of whether they took place in a care home or not, are connected by an embodied, intuitive and intimate relationship between people and things. By emphasising the nature of being in relationships, this type of performance transcends physical ability, cognitive capacity, or a formal arts training, offering an opportunity to be present in the here and now. As Anne Basting puts it, 'Art-making gives us a way of being in relationships... as artists, as teachers, as learners, as human beings on the journey to old age ourselves, this is all we can hope for' (2016, p. 163).

Note

1. In 2019, for example, the National Theatre in London cast Sarah Gordy, an actor with Down's Syndrome, in *Jellyfish*, a production about a woman with Downs Syndrome and her relationship with a neurotypical man. In the same year, the National Theatre of Scotland became the first of the UK's national theatres to open a residency scheme for neurodiverse artists.

References

Basting, A, (2016). In Basting A, Towey, M, and Rose, E, (eds). *The Penelope Project: An Arts-Based Odyssey to Change Elder Care.* Iowa: University of Iowa Press.

Begault, M., Hodson, K., & Langford, S. (2017). *Magic Me's Artist Residencies in Care Homes.* Retrieved September 1, 2019, from https://magicme.co.uk/wp-content/uploads/2018/03/Artists-Residences-in-Care-Homes-report-WEB-low.pdf

Hargrave, M. (2017). Dance with a Stranger. Torque Show's 'Intimacy' (2014) and the Experience of Vulnerability in Performance and Spectatorship. In A. O'Grady (Ed.), *Risk, Participation and Performance Practice: Critical Vulnerabilities in a Precarious World.* Basingstoke: Palgrave Macmillan.

Kontos, P., Miller, K., & Kontos, A. (2017). Relational Citizenship: Supporting Embodied Selfhood and Relationality in Dementia Care. *Sociology of Health and Illness, 39*(2), 182–198.

Jackson, S. (2011). *Social Works: Performing Art, Supporting Publics.* Oxon: Routledge.

LaBelle, B. (2006). *Background Noise: Perspectives in Sound Art.* New York: Continuum.

Postscript. A Cultural Response to Care after Covid-19

Bradford, 2020

It is December 2020 and like so many others, my work and family life has changed radically since the outbreak of Covid-19. While news of a vaccine has offered some much-needed hope, there is a great deal of uncertainty about the long-term impact of the pandemic. One thing that feels likely is that Covid-19 it will significantly change the way in which we look after people in care homes and the opportunities to bring arts practices into care spaces. The priority for care homes is protecting staff and residents, and the re-introduction of artists is something that will have to be negotiated safely and gradually. When artists do return, creative approaches may look different. Many of the practices outlined in this book such as tactility, object work, singing and hand to body contact may need to be re-imagined.

In response to social distancing restrictions, many practitioners are finding new ways to maintain relationships with care home residents during lockdown. Artists whose work was previously characterised by intimate encounters inside care homes have adapted their practice, creating work virtually, digitally, outdoors, up against windows, and through the post. In Milwaukee, *Timeslips* practitioners have organised, among other initiatives, the exchange of creative postcards which share 'a hopeful poem, a

N. Hatton, *Performance and Dementia*,
https://doi.org/10.1007/978-3-030-51077-0

drawing, or a 'beautiful question'. In Berlin, a group of 'socially distanced clowns' have taken to performing in courtyards outside residents' bedrooms. In London, the intergenerational arts charity Magic Me have sent creative care packages to residents each month, and there are numerous stories emerging of residents being entertained by singers, dancers and poets outside doors and windows.

As well as demonstrating the commitment that artists have to maintaining relationships with care home residents, these small-scale interventions demonstrate the possibilities of a more physically distanced but equally as creative response to care. As artists learn more about the possibilities of 'Zoom Theatre', adapting theatre for podcasts, creating digital content and live streaming performances, there is the potential to bring a broader range of high-quality theatrical experiences to residents. This of course, requires technology such as tablets and a reliable internet connection—something which a lot of care homes do not yet have, but the impetus to fund technology in care homes, both as a means of social contact and access to creative activities, has never been greater. By exploring the perimeters of socially distanced live work in care homes, performance practitioners and residents may experience a range of new spaces such as courtyards, car parks and gardens, as creative spaces. With imagination, there is also the potential to create micro creative spaces indoors. A care home in York has been among the first to install a Covid visitor pod with an airtight glass screen and an intercom system to allow residents to meet their loved ones again. Strange as this might have sounded before the outbreak, inventions such as this may enable new creative spaces to emerge, and for artists, care staff and residents to interact in new ways.

These examples of practice offer a glimpse of how relationships between people and things may still be nurtured and maintained artfully in the context of social distancing and other infection control measures. We don't have to look far for examples of community solidarity during Covid, and it is, in many cases, creative acts of care—the making of music on balconies, the curation of care packages for neighbours, the homemade rainbows for NHS workers—that has brought people closer together. Socially distanced relationships can never replace the sense of connection that comes with physical contact, but the pandemic has, perhaps, taught us something new about the art of care. As we look to heal and rebuild communities of care after Covid, the notion of interdependence has never been more critical. The hope and connections that have emerged during the pandemic reiterate the importance of the arts in building and sustaining mutually caring relationships—both inside and outside of care settings.

Index[1]

[1] Note: Page numbers followed by 'n' refer to notes.

N. Hatton, *Performance and Dementia*,
https://doi.org/10.1007/978-3-030-51077-0

The manufacturer's authorised representative in the EU is Springer Nature Customer Service Centre GmbH, Europaplatz 3, 69115 Heidelberg, Germany. If you have any concerns regarding our products, please contact ProductSafety@springernature.com

Printed and bound by CPI Group (UK) Ltd, Croydon, CR0 4YY
30/09/2026
02225453-0003